AMA
AMERICAN
MEDICAL
ASSOCIATION

BOY'S GUIDE TO BECOMING A TEEN

Amy B. Middleman, MD, MSEd, MPH, Medical Editor

Kate Gruenwald Pfeifer, LCSW, Writer

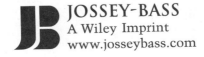

JOSSEY-BASS
A Wiley Imprint
www.josseybass.com

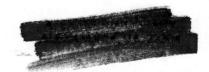

This book is printed on acid-free paper. ∞

Copyright © 2006 by The American Medical Association. All rights reserved.

Published by Jossey-Bass
A Wiley Imprint
989 Market Street, San Francisco, CA 94103-1741

Developed by Nancy Hall, Inc.
Illustrations by Brie Spangler

The recommendations and information in this book are appropriate in most cases and current as of the date of publication. For more specific information about a medical condition, the AMA suggests that you consult a physician.

No part of this publication may be reproduced, stored in a retrieval system, or transmitted in any form or by any means, electronic, mechanical, photocopying, recording, scanning, or otherwise, except as permitted under Section 107 or 108 of the 1976 United States Copyright Act, without either the prior written permission of the Publisher, or authorization through payment of the appropriate per-copy fee to the Copyright Clearance Center, Inc., 222 Rosewood Drive, Danvers, MA 01923, 978-750-8400, fax 978-646-8600, or on the Web at www.copyright.com. Requests to the Publisher for permission should be addressed to the Permissions Department, John Wiley & Sons, Inc., 111 River Street, Hoboken, NJ 07030, 201-748-6011, fax 201-748-6008, or online at http://www.wiley.com/go/permissions.

Limit of Liability/Disclaimer of Warranty: While the publisher and the author have used their best efforts in preparing this book, they make no representations or warranties with respect to the accuracy or completeness of the contents of this book and specifically disclaim any implied warranties of merchantability or fitness for a particular purpose. No warranty may be created or extended by sales representatives or written sales materials. The advice and strategies contained herein may not be suitable for your situation. You should consult with a professional where appropriate. Neither the publisher nor the author shall be liable for any loss of profit or any other commercial damages, including but not limited to special, incidental, consequential, or other damages.

Readers should be aware that Internet Web sites offered as citations and/or sources for further information may have changed or disappeared between the time this was written and when it is read.

Permission is given for individual classroom teachers to reproduce the pages and illustrations for classroom use. Reproduction of these materials for an entire school system is strictly forbidden.

Jossey-Bass books and products are available through most bookstores. To contact Jossey-Bass directly, call our Customer Care Department within the U.S. at 800-956-7739, outside the U.S. at 317-572-3986, or fax 317-572-4002.

Jossey-Bass also publishes its books in a variety of electronic formats. Some content that appears in print may not be available in electronic books.

Library of Congress Cataloging-in-Publication Data
American Medical Association boy's guide to becoming a teen.
     p. cm.
  Includes index.
  ISBN-13: 978-0-7879-8343-7 (pbk. : alk. paper)
  ISBN-10: 0-7879-8343-8 (pbk. : alk. paper)
  1. Puberty—Juvenile literature. 2. Teenage boys—Physiology—Juvenile literature.
  I. Title: Boys' guide to becoming a teen. II. American Medical Association.
  RJ143.A43 2006
  613'.04233—dc22

                                                        2005034809

Printed in the United States of America

first edition

PB Printing 10 9 8 7 6 5 4 3 2 1

FOREWORD......................................

This is a very important, very exciting time in your life as you go through so many changes on your way to becoming an adult. Along with the transformation your body is undergoing, many other things in your life are changing, too. For example, your relationships with your parents and your friends may be different now than when you were younger, and people may treat you differently. Also, the way you look at things is probably not the same as it used to be. Of course, you have lots of questions. We at the American Medical Association have created this book to give you the answers to many of those questions—information that can help you grow up healthy and happy. You can also turn to your parents, your doctor, and other trusted adults whenever you need more information, guidance, or help. With more facts, you can make even better decisions to keep yourself safe.

In this book, you will learn how to deal with common concerns boys have, such as body changes, acne, and relationships. You will learn why it's so important, even at your age, to eat a healthy diet and to be physically active. This book also discusses many of the issues that may soon be facing you or your friends, including how to resist pressure from other kids to drink alcohol, smoke cigarettes, use drugs, or start becoming sexually active.

The handy glossary at the back of the book explains some of the medical terms used in the book. Also at the end of the book, you'll find a list of helpful Web sites to go to for more information.

We at the AMA wish you good health on your journey into adulthood!

American Medical Association

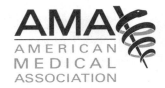

AMERICAN
MEDICAL
ASSOCIATION

Michael D. Maves, MD, MBA	Executive Vice President, Chief Executive Officer
Robert A. Musacchio, PhD	Senior Vice President, Publishing and Business Services
Anthony J. Frankos	Vice President, Business Products
Mary Lou White	Executive Director, Editorial and Operations
Amy B. Middleman, MD, MSEd, MPH	Medical Editor
Donna Kotulak	Managing Editor
Mary Ann Albanese	Art Editor
Arthur Elster, MD	Director, Division of Medicine and Public Health, AMA
Missy Fleming, PhD	Program Director, Child and Adolescent Health, AMA
Mary R. Casek, MAT	Educational Consultant

CONTENTS

CHAPTER ONE
Welcome to Puberty

If you're reading this, it's probably because you're about to become a teenager. There are a lot of great things about becoming a teenager. You get taller, bigger, and stronger. You get better at many of the things you enjoy doing, like playing a musical instrument, drawing, or being on the soccer team. You begin to have more freedom—to go more places and do more things with your friends. You may start dating. You may even get your first job and have your own money to spend in ways that *you* want to spend it. These things all make becoming a teenager an exciting time in your life.

This book will help you know what to expect as your body and mind go through some pretty major changes. It will answer most, if not all, of the many questions you are likely to have as you go through puberty. Of course, it's also a very good idea to talk to your parents, other family members, a doctor or nurse, or other trusted adults about any concerns you have.

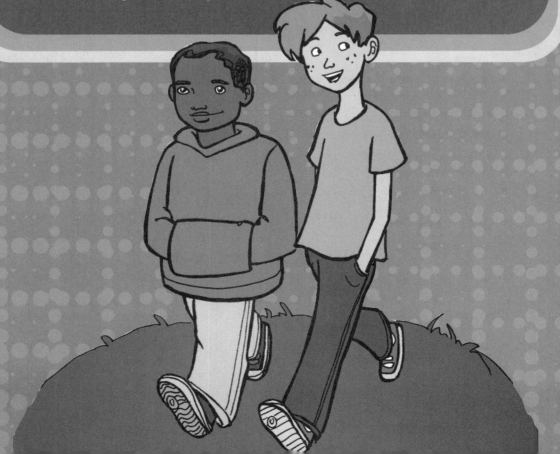

Hey! Don't be shy about asking questions.
Remember that all adults were once as young as
you and went through the same changes!

What is puberty?

Puberty is the process that your body goes through as you grow from a child to an adult. During puberty, your body and mind change in many ways. Puberty is also the time when your voice gets deeper and you start to look less like a kid and more like a grown-up.

Some of the changes you will notice as you go through puberty:

- You get taller.
- Your shoulders get wider.
- Your muscles get bigger.
- You grow hair in new places.
- Your voice gets deeper and lower.

In addition to these physical changes, you might notice other changes in yourself. Your relationships with your family and friends might change, too. It's not always easy to go through so many changes so quickly. Puberty can be exciting, confusing, scary, or no big deal—each reaction is perfectly normal.

Does this ever happen to you?

- Your body seems to look and feel different every week.
- Your voice cracks when *you* answer a question in class and you hope no one noticed.
- You spend more time with new friends than with old ones.

What is adolescence?

Adolescence is the period of time between the end of childhood development and adulthood. This period starts at about age 11 or 12 and continues through the late teen years and early 20s. Adolescence is a time of change—learning who you are and who you want to become—and it includes the path to getting there.

How long does puberty last?

Puberty generally starts sometime between the ages of 9 and 14. For many boys, it takes about 5 to 6 years to go through all the different stages of puberty. But every boy is unique and will go through puberty in his own way and at his own pace.

You might notice that some boys in your class seem to be finishing the last stage of puberty while other boys seem to still be in the first stage. This is normal, because there is no exact timetable for puberty that everyone follows.

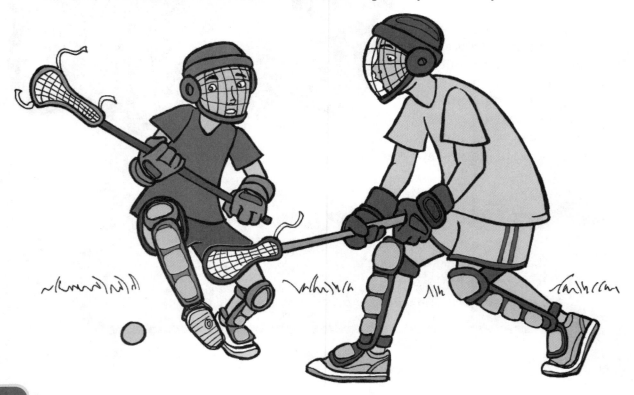

How should I feel about puberty?

Different boys have different feelings about starting puberty. Some boys can't wait to see changes in their body. They feel ready to look and act more like an adult. Other boys are not quite so ready. They're still interested in their old toys and games and are comfortable still being a kid. And some boys alternate between feeling ready and feeling not quite so ready to move on. Whichever of these ways you feel is normal.

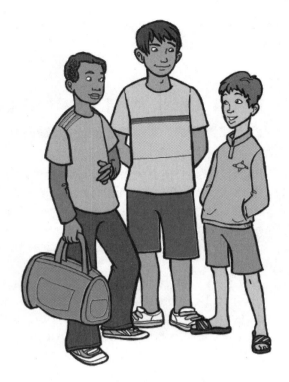

It can be hard to be one of the first boys in class to go through puberty. You may feel that people expect you to act older than you really are. Or some kids may tease you about your facial hair or having to use deodorant before everyone else.

Whether you go through puberty early or late, you're going to go through it in your own way. Try to focus more on enjoying it than worrying about when it will happen!

It can also be hard to start puberty later than your friends. It can seem like people still see you as a younger kid. Or you might be teased for being shorter or smaller than other kids.

The fact is, boys start puberty at different ages. There is no "normal" age for puberty to begin. Also, some boys may start puberty earlier than other boys but end puberty later. Knowing that, if you still feel worried about starting puberty, talk to your parents or your doctor. Ask your father when he started puberty. Chances are that you will go through puberty at a similar age as, and in a similar way to, your dad.

Why will my feelings change during puberty?

Puberty is a time when many boys become more self-conscious. You may find that you begin to worry more than before about how others see you. You may start to compare yourself to your friends, noticing that some of them look older than you and that some seem better at things you find important, like playing sports or getting attention from other people.

You may notice that you and your parents don't always seem as close as you used to be. You may not want your parents to know as much about your life as you were willing to share when you were younger. Your parents might ask you if there is something wrong because you may be more quiet or keep to yourself more than usual.

Does this ever happen to you?

One minute you may feel like a kid who wants to play and the next minute you feel more grown-up, wanting more freedom and independence.

Puberty is also a time when you may begin to think about the world and your place in it. You might decide to pursue some special interests. You may start to read newspapers or watch the news and learn about some issues in the world that concern you. You may even notice something about your school or your neighborhood that troubles you. Can you make a difference, and, if so, how? These are all normal feelings and questions for teenagers.

The changes you are experiencing occur for many reasons. One reason is that your hormones are changing. *Hormones* are chemicals that are responsible for many processes in the body, including growth and development, and even mood. During puberty your way of thinking also changes as your brain further develops.

Another reason you may be feeling different is that your life is changing. You may have switched schools, starting middle school or junior high. You may feel more pressures and responsibilities as you get older. You may have made new friends, started thinking about dating, or gone through a family change like a divorce or moving to a new town. These are all big changes and they are likely to affect the way you feel.

If you have special needs or a long-term illness, whether or not others know about it, going through the many changes of puberty can sometimes be challenging. You're certainly not alone. Whenever you find things especially difficult, you'll feel better if you express your feelings to your parents, your doctor, the school nurse, a counselor, or another adult you trust. It can also be helpful to talk to other kids your age—you'll quickly realize that you all have a lot in common.

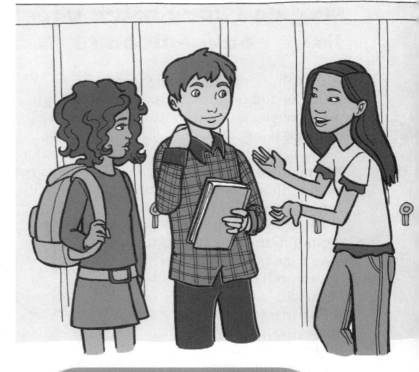

Some Ways You Can Make a Difference

- Help an elderly neighbor.
- Read to a younger child.
- Organize a fundraiser for a worthy cause.
- Stop an act of bullying.
- When you're old enough, volunteer at a local hospital, nursing home, soup kitchen, or animal shelter.

Why do I care more about what I look like? I never used to think about it.

You might notice that how you look seems more important as you become a teenager. You overhear girls talking about which boys they think are cute and see them giggle as you walk by. You may begin to wonder if they think *you're* cute and if any of that giggling has to do with you.

You might start comparing yourself to other boys in your school and neighborhood. Some of them might seem taller and more muscular than you. You may think, "I hate getting changed for gym in the locker room. I'm the only boy who hasn't started to grow underarm hair yet. I still look like a kid!" Or "I'm one of the shortest boys in my grade—people never seem to pay attention to me!" These are common ways that boys your age compare themselves to others.

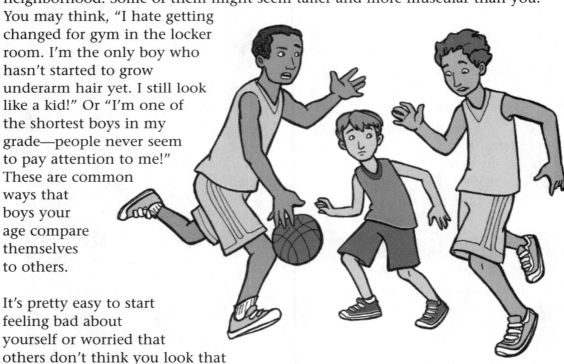

It's pretty easy to start feeling bad about yourself or worried that others don't think you look that great. The bottom line is that nobody has the perfect body, or face, or set of muscles. Not even those guys you see in fitness magazines! Although it's normal to find things about yourself that you want to change, try not to be too critical of yourself. Constantly putting yourself down does nothing but make you feel bad. Try to remind yourself of the things you like about yourself when you start to feel bad. Here's an example: "I may be shorter than most boys, but I'm really funny and easy to talk to." Or, "I may be smaller than most of the other kids, but they're always asking me for help with math." If you're having a hard time finding those good qualities in yourself, ask someone you trust—a good friend or a parent or another adult you look up to. You might be surprised to hear how many good things the people who know you see in you!

Did you know that the photographs of guys you see in fitness magazines and ads have been touched up quite a bit to make them look more muscular and to make their skin look more clear? These men would look very different if you saw them in person. They would look more like everyone else—not perfect!

What is happening to my voice lately? One minute it sounds squeaky and the next it sounds so deep.

During puberty, your *vocal cords* grow longer and wider. Your voice box (which doctors call the *larynx*) grows too. This change to your vocal cords causes your voice to get lower and deeper, making you sound more like an adult than a child. But don't expect this change to happen overnight!

When your voice box grows, you may notice it as a lump in the middle of your throat. This is usually referred to as an *Adam's apple*. Most boys have an Adam's apple, while most girls don't because their voice box doesn't grow as much as a boy's.

While it's happening, your voice might seem to go up and down. It can sound high-pitched and squeaky one minute and deep and scratchy the next. This is normal. But don't worry—the squeaking will stop and your voice will even out at the lower range.

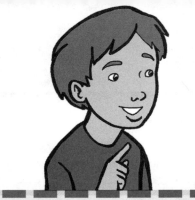

REAL BOYS, REAL FEELINGS

I play on a hockey team. My dad wants me to try out for the baseball team because he used to play it. I don't know how to tell him that I just want to play ice hockey. Age 11

My dad yells at my soccer coach during games and makes me want to crawl in a hole. It makes me not want to play sports. I have to say something to him. Age 10

I'm skinny and I want to bulk up, so a friend told me about steroids. My dad found out about it and printed out a list of all the scary things steroids could do to me. I don't want to deal with those problems, so I'll stick to push-ups and lifting weights. Age 12

I go to dance class with my older sister. One of my friends found out and says I'm a sissy. I like the classes and I like to dance so I don't care what he says. Age 10

One of the guys at school found some pills. I don't want to "rat" but I'm scared that some of my friends will take the pills with him. Age 12

My parents want me to stop playing so many video games, but it's my favorite thing to do. My grades are good. I don't see why I can't spend my time how I want. Age 10

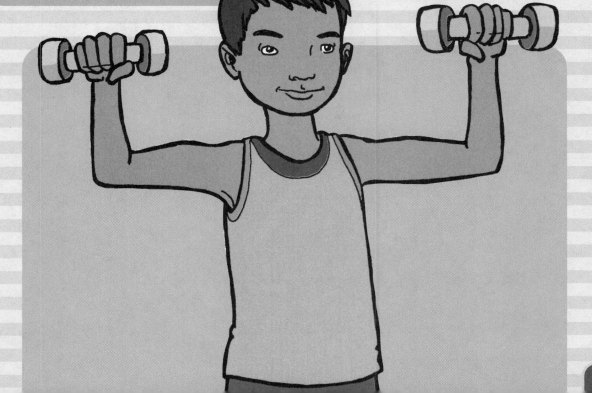

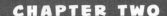

CHAPTER TWO
Eating, Exercise, and a Healthy Weight

Most teenage boys worry about what their body looks like. Everyone wants to look good. But what does looking good mean to you? Do you want to be big and muscular? Or would you prefer to be thin and lean? Do you worry about being chubby? Or do you struggle with feeling you're skinny? No matter what body type you have—or want—there are certain things you should know that can help you stay healthy.

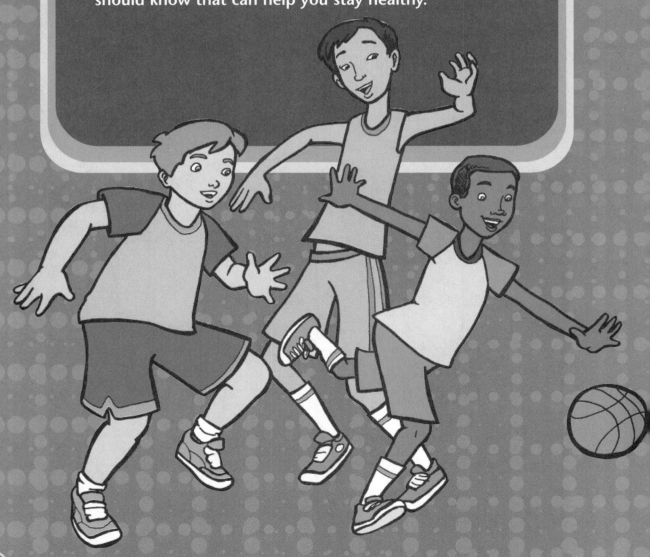

Why do I need to pay attention to what I eat?

It's especially important to be a healthy eater at this time in your life. Your brain and body need nutritious food at regular times so you can learn, grow, and be active. If you eat too many of the wrong kinds of foods, your body isn't getting the vitamins, minerals, and other nutrients it needs to function well and keep you healthy. Foods like french fries, 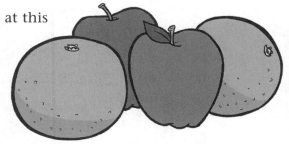 chips, sugary soft drinks and fruit drinks have lots of *calories* but few of the nutrients your body needs. Also be aware that fruit drinks are not so good for you because they contain a lot of sugar and little else besides water; it's much healthier to eat an orange or an apple or other fruit than to drink fruit juice.

How often do I need to eat?

Eating frequently is important. You should be eating three meals a day, with one or two snacks in between. Nutritious food enables your body and muscles to grow and develop.

Have you ever noticed that it can be really hard to concentrate in class if you've skipped breakfast? Your brain does not function at its best when you go for long periods without eating.

Does this ever happen to you?

When you skip breakfast:
- You get a headache in the middle of the morning.
- You do badly on a test.
- You fall asleep in class.
- You have trouble paying attention to the teacher.

Many boys find that they are hungrier than ever as they begin puberty. Your parents might even start complaining that they can't keep the refrigerator stocked because you're eating so much! This is normal. Your body is getting ready to go through a growth spurt (more on that in chapter 3) and it needs more food than usual to fuel that growth spurt.

Some boys don't feel very hungry and aren't interested in eating three meals and one snack a day. If this sounds like you, talk to your doctor or the school nurse. Tell him or her that you need help coming up with some ideas for making eating more appealing to you.

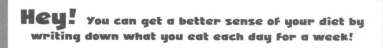

Hey! You can get a better sense of your diet by writing down what you eat each day for a week!

What kinds of foods should I be eating?

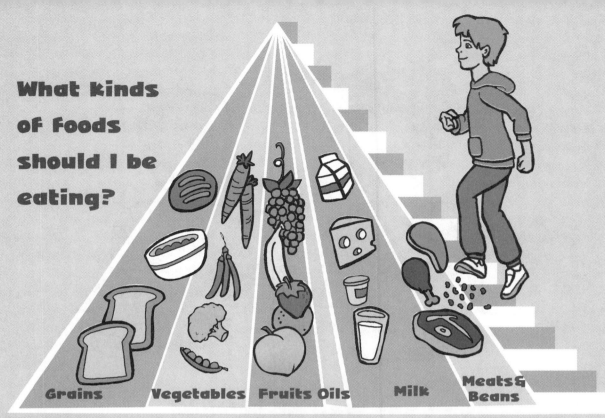

Grains | Vegetables | Fruits Oils | Milk | Meats & Beans

Grains	Vegetables	Fruits	Milk	Meats & Beans
Eat whole-grain breads, cereals, and pastas — they're better for you than non-whole-grain foods!	Choose a colorful variety of vegetables to make sure you get a broad range of vitamins!	Grab a piece of fruit when you want a sweet snack— it has lots more nutrition than juice!	Most dairy products are high in calcium, which helps build and maintain strong bones!	Choose lean meat whenever possible. Chicken, turkey, and fish are great choices!
*Eat about 6 ounces of grains a day. An ounce equals 1 slice of bread, 1 cup of cereal, or 1/2 cup of pasta	*Eat about 2½ cups of vegetables a day.	*Eat about 1½ cups of fruit a day.	*Eat about 3 cups of dairy foods a day.	*Eat about 5 ounces of meat and beans a day. Three ounces of meat is the size of a deck of cards.

Oils: Oils from fish, nuts, and liquid oils (such as olive, soybean, or canola) are good for you in moderation!

Use this food guide pyramid to learn what types of food you should eat. You can see that you should be eating a certain number of servings of foods from each category every day, with more servings of some kinds of foods than of others. For example, you should be eating more fruits and vegetables, whole-grain breads and cereals, and low-fat dairy products like skim milk, and less sugary and fatty foods such as soft drinks, candy, cookies, and chips.

*Portion recommendations are based on an 1,800-calorie diet.

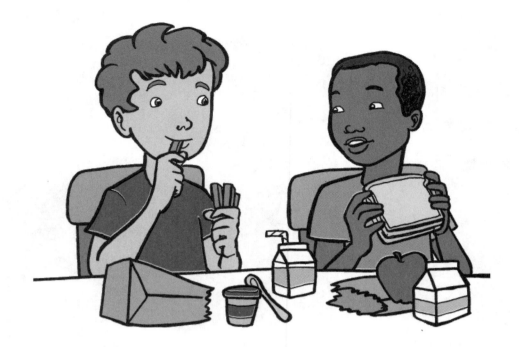

How can I eat well at school?

You might notice that you have more food choices in your school cafeteria as you enter middle school. But not all of these choices are healthy. Many school cafeterias offer high-calorie, high-fat, sugary, low-nutrient foods such as fried foods and sugary snack foods and soft drinks and juices. You need to be careful about what you choose!

If you eat and drink a lot of these kinds of foods, you may find yourself becoming overweight. If you look carefully around your school cafeteria, you should be able to find some better options. Increasing numbers of schools are offering more nutritious choices such as soup, salads, and fruit, as well as sandwiches and wraps. Choose these kinds of foods and, instead of sugary soft drinks and fruit juices, drink water and low-fat or fat-free milk.

A healthy option is to bring a packed lunch or snack from home. This way, you can make sure you're eating something that's both nutritious and something you really like. Some good snack choices from home include your favorite sandwich, some fruit, some cut-up veggies, or pretzels.

What if I want to try out a different diet, like vegetarian?

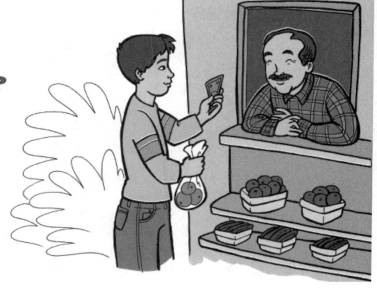

Because of your age and the importance of getting enough *nutrients* for growth, you should talk to your doctor before you make any changes in your eating habits. *Vegetarians* need to focus even more than other people on eating a balanced diet. Restricting whole food groups from your diet can be harmful to your health, especially at your age. If you eliminate meat and poultry from your diet, you need to add other *protein* sources because protein is essential for your body to develop and grow properly. Good non-meat protein sources include kidney beans and other beans, eggs, low-fat milk and cheese, nuts, and tofu.

> THERE ARE 3 TYPES OF VEGETARIANS:
> ◆ *Lacto-ovo-vegetarians* do not eat meats, but their diets do include milk and eggs.
> ◆ *Lacto-vegetarians* do not eat meats or eggs, but their diets do include milk and dairy products.
> ◆ *Vegans* do not eat meats, eggs, or dairy.

Your doctor may recommend that you meet with a dietitian; a *dietitian* is a trained health professional who teaches people how to eat healthfully. The dietitian can tell you about different food combinations you should eat to make sure you are getting the right amounts of *vitamins*, *minerals*, and other nutrients to stay healthy. But just to be safe, it's a good idea to also take a daily multivitamin/mineral supplement.

Is exercise important at my age?

Exercise is just as important as eating a healthy diet—at any age. You should be doing something physical every day for at least 1 hour. Exercise can include activities as varied as walking to school, jogging, riding your bike, shooting baskets, or playing on a sports team or in the marching band.

It's also important to get different kinds of exercise. The three types of exercise are aerobic, strengthening, and flexibility. Aerobic exercises—such as walking, jogging, and bike riding—use the large muscles in your body and get your heart rate up. Strengthening exercises—such as push-ups, crunches, and lifting weights—make your muscles bigger and stronger. Flexibility exercises—like stretching—make your muscles and joints flexible and help prevent injuries. It's a good idea to do stretches for a few minutes before and especially after you do aerobic exercises such as jogging and running.

The most important thing to consider when it comes to exercise is to have fun! Try different activities and alternate between them so you don't get bored. That way, you'll be exercising and toning different parts of your body.

How do I avoid sports injuries?

The most important step you can take to avoid injuries is to always use the proper equipment for the activity. For example, wear a helmet if you are bike riding, skiing, snowboarding, rollerblading, or skateboarding. If you're playing a team sport, always wear the proper equipment, like a mouth guard, jock strap, cup, shin guards, or protective eyewear. Safety equipment is always your best defense against injury.

Of course, even with the proper equipment, it is still possible to get hurt. Report an injury as soon as you realize that something is wrong. Ignoring it can make it worse. If you're playing on a team, tell your coach as soon as you're injured. It's also very important to let your doctor know about any injuries or symptoms you are experiencing. He or she will be able to tell you how to treat the injury and will also tell you how to avoid the injury in the future.

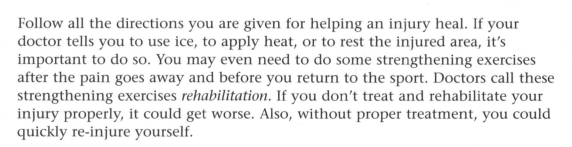

Follow all the directions you are given for helping an injury heal. If your doctor tells you to use ice, to apply heat, or to rest the injured area, it's important to do so. You may even need to do some strengthening exercises after the pain goes away and before you return to the sport. Doctors call these strengthening exercises *rehabilitation*. If you don't treat and rehabilitate your injury properly, it could get worse. Also, without proper treatment, you could quickly re-injure yourself.

My parents keep bugging me about how much time I spend playing video games. What's the big deal?

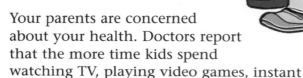

Your parents are concerned about your health. Doctors report that the more time kids spend watching TV, playing video games, instant messaging, surfing the Internet, and just plain sitting around, the less physically fit they are—and the more likely they are to be overweight. Of course, these activities are fun for preteens and teens. But doctors recommend that kids spend no more than 1 or 2 hours a day doing them.

If you spend more time than that playing with electronics, you are not allowing enough time for other, more constructive activities, such as homework, reading, and physical exercise.

So, to keep yourself healthy and to get your parents to stop reminding you, turn off the TV, shut down the computer, and go outside and be physical. You're sure to feel better if you do!

What changes can I expect to see in my body?

Your body will change a lot during puberty. You will become taller, stronger, and more muscular. Your shoulders will become broader. Your muscles will become thicker because your body is now making more of the male hormone testosterone. If you want, you can make your muscles even more defined by exercising.

Is it okay for kids my age to lift weights?

The answer is usually yes, but you don't want to rush it. You need to talk to your doctor about it to make sure your body is ready for weight-lifting exercises and it is safe for you to do. The doctor can also tell you about injury risks and discuss your goals. Before you begin weight training, it's important to work with a professional trainer or coach who can show you how to perform the exercises properly to avoid injuries.

You should start slow and small, using lighter weights at first to make sure you learn the correct, safe techniques for each exercise. Then you can slowly build up to heavier weights, under the trainer's or coach's supervision.

Don't Overdo It!

Working out more than three times a week or two days in a row or with too-heavy weights won't help you get stronger faster—but will increase your risk of injury. Because you are still growing, you should not be doing power lifting or body building. Also keep in mind that strength-building exercises are just one part of your overall fitness plan; you also need to do aerobic and flexibility exercises.

How do I get the body I want?

Like everyone, teenage boys have all sorts of body shapes and sizes. Some boys are naturally tall and skinny, some are naturally muscular, and others tend to be rounder. Your body type is largely determined by *heredity*. This means that you will probably have a body type similar to that of other people in your family. For example, if people in your family tend to be on the short side and muscular, chances are that you will be too.

It makes sense that your body type is determined by heredity—after all, so are your hair color, nose shape, and other traits. You may not be thrilled with one or another characteristic that you inherited, but it's likely that you are very happy with many of your other traits!

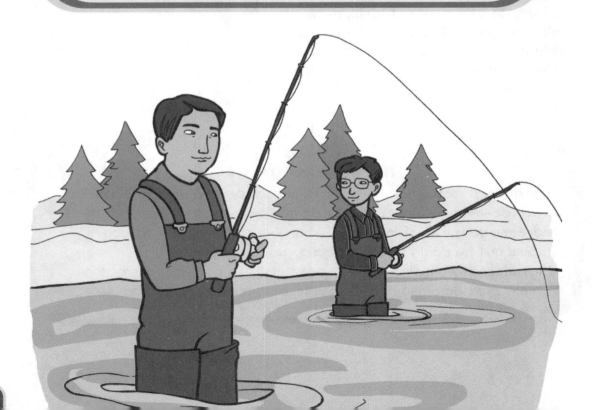

What am I supposed to weigh?

Your weight will change a lot during puberty as you get taller. This is because your body is growing and changing all the time. Some boys will put on weight more quickly, while other boys may have a harder time gaining weight. Your doctor can let you know what is a normal weight range for your height and body type.

What do I do if I think I'm overweight?

Eating a healthy diet is always a good idea for teenagers, even if you are overweight. You need to eat regularly to grow taller and to develop muscles. If you're worried about your weight, talk to your parents and then to your doctor. He or she can help you come up with ways to choose healthy foods. Your doctor can also help you learn how to eat sensible portions of foods to help you get to a healthy weight.

Boys need a lot of calories to fuel their rapid growth during puberty. To help you reach a healthy weight, your doctor may recommend that you get more physically active; the more active you are, the more calories your body burns and the more fit and toned your body will be!

27

What do I do if I think I'm underweight?

If you think you might need to gain weight, talk to your parents and then to your doctor. You may be thin because you are going through your growth spurt and have gotten taller but haven't gained as much weight yet. Or you may be in a family that tends to be thin naturally.

If you want to gain some weight and the doctor thinks it's okay for you to do so, you might try eating more often, by adding an additional healthy snack or two between meals. Whatever you do, don't eat fatty or sugary junk foods as a way to gain weight because too much fat and sugar can be harmful to your health.

What if I'm unhappy with my body?

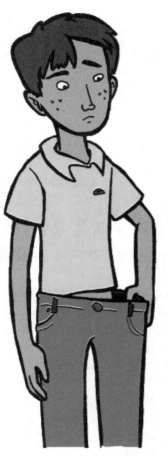

Everyone has times when they don't feel so good about their body. But if you notice that you're having negative thoughts about your body *most* of the time, this can be the sign of a problem.

Some boys might try to restrict their eating in order to lose weight. Other boys might start eating uncontrollably and then feel bad about it afterward. Some boys might find themselves exercising for hours every day, trying to achieve the perfect body.

None of these approaches is healthy. If you notice that you or a friend is doing any of the things described above, get help. Talk to your parents, your doctor, or a school counselor or other trusted adult immediately.

What are anabolic steroids?

Steroids are hormones the body produces to help your body deal with stress and to promote growth and development. Some steroids are prescribed by doctors to treat medical problems. *Anabolic steroids* are versions of the male hormone testosterone, which is responsible for male characteristics. These drugs can be taken in the form of pills, powder, or injection. Most anabolic steroids are illegal and are banned by professional sports organizations and, when used for non-medical reasons, are condemned by doctors.

Some athletes take anabolic steroids to make their muscles bigger and stronger. But they are taking a big health risk. Anabolic steroids can make your testicles shrink and your breasts grow, and they can make you infertile (unable to have children). In extreme cases, they can lead to an increased risk of a heart attack or cancer. Anabolic steroids can also cause acne, oily hair, high blood pressure, hair loss, and mood swings. Anabolic steroids can be addictive; some young people who have used them and tried to stop have developed severe depression and become suicidal.

Steroidal supplements sold at some health food stores and gyms are also anabolic steroids. Because these supplements are not regulated by the government, no one knows for sure what harmful effects they could have on the body. Teenagers should *never* use any type of anabolic steroid.

Guess What!

Athletes who take anabolic steroids may want to be winners—but they're actually losers!

CHAPTER THREE
Your Height

Most boys look forward to growing taller during puberty. Some will grow very tall during this time. Big increases in height are called *growth spurts*. During a growth spurt, you will grow several inches in a pretty short period of time.

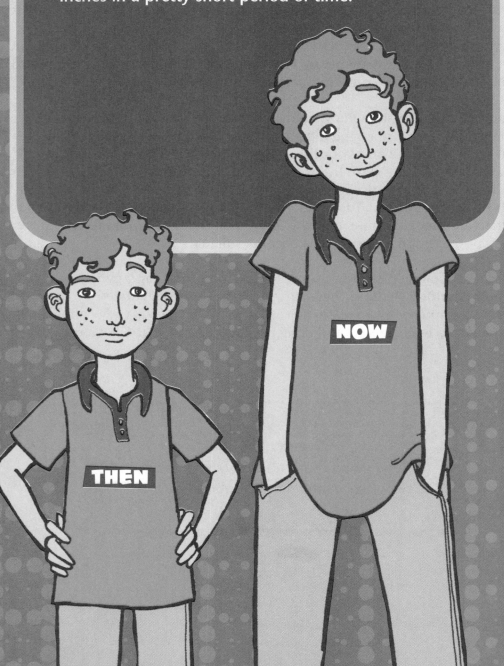

THEN

NOW

When will I start to get taller?

The average boy grows fastest at around ages 14 and 15 and usually finishes growing at around age 20. But keep in mind that these are averages. Just like every other part of puberty, there is no way to predict exactly when *you* will start going through *your* growth spurt. Some boys will start earlier and others will start later.

It can be difficult being the tallest boy in the class, just as it can be tough being the shortest. Teenage boys worry a lot about their height. Although thinking about your height is normal, try not to stress out about it.

How much will I grow?

When you were younger, you grew

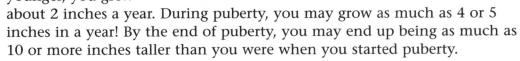

about 2 inches a year. During puberty, you may grow as much as 4 or 5 inches in a year! By the end of puberty, you may end up being as much as 10 or more inches taller than you were when you started puberty.

The average height for men in the United States is 5 feet 10 inches. But look at the men you know and you will see that their heights differ quite a lot. Some men reach a height well over 6 feet, while others are much shorter than 5 feet 10 inches.

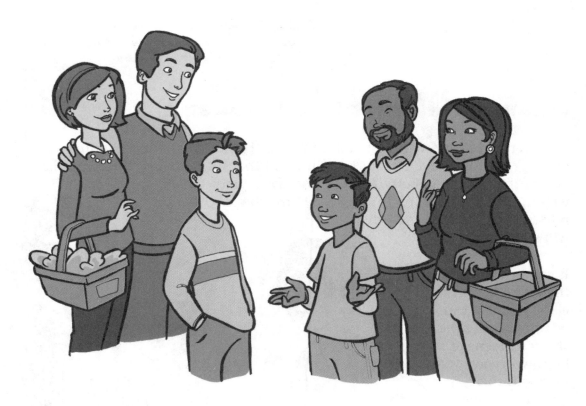

Your height is based mostly on heredity. If members of your family are mostly on the tall side, it's likely that you will also be tall. If most people in your family are short, it's likely that you too will be on the shorter side.

For fun, try the following formula to get an estimate of how tall you might be. First, find out the height in inches of both of your parents. (Don't forget that you have to multiply the number of feet by 12 to turn feet into inches; so if your dad is 6 feet tall, he is 6 x 12 = 72 inches tall.) Then add 5 inches to your mom's height and add this number to your dad's height. Divide the sum by 2. Although there is no way to precisely predict a person's future height, this formula can give you a measurement to think about. After all, it *is* possible that you will end up being much taller or much shorter than both of your parents— or anyone else in your family!

When will I stop growing?

Most boys finish growing taller by their late teens or early 20s. This does not mean that *your* growth spurt will last that many years! You'll probably grow quite a bit in a couple of years, and then your growth will start to slow down again.

Why are so many girls taller than boys in middle school?

Girls tend to start puberty earlier than boys, which means they also start their growth spurt sooner. It's common for girls in middle school to be taller than the boys in their grade. This can be awkward for both girls and boys. The taller girls may feel self-conscious and some of the boys may feel embarrassed. Remember that growing in height is another normal part of puberty. Because boys have more time to grow before they start their growth spurt and grow a bit more in height than girls during the growth spurt, they usually end up taller by the time high school is over. Always be kind to other kids no matter how tall or short they are. No one has control over his or her height; if someone is bothered by it, teasing can make him or her uncomfortable.

Why do my feet seem so big lately?

Certain parts of your body may grow earlier and faster than other parts. You may notice that your feet seem to be growing quickly all of a sudden. You may even get a new pair of sneakers and outgrow them before you've had a chance to wear them!

The bones in the hands and feet usually grow first during a growth spurt. Then the arms and legs grow longer, and finally the spine. At the end of your growth spurt, your chest and shoulders will expand. Having some parts of your body grow at different times can occasionally make you feel awkward. But don't worry—it will all even out in time and you'll get used to your new body!

What if I'm really unhappy with my height?

Men in our society feel a lot of pressure about their height. Many boys think they need to be tall and strong in order to get attention. Or they worry that they won't be successful if they're short. But this is far from the reality. Just look around at the men you know—you'll see that height has nothing to do with getting a good job, being smart, being respected, falling in love, or being good at sports.

Also keep in mind that you have no control over your height. So try not to waste too much time thinking about it. Instead, focus on things you *do* have control over. You want to be more popular? Think of ways that you can start conversations or make people laugh. You want to get a good job some day? Study hard and keep your grades up. You want to be a star in the school play, make the soccer team, or play in the school band? Work hard, practice, and focus on improving your skills.

Taller boys also worry about their height. If you're tall, you may feel self-conscious about it and wish that you weren't so much taller than everyone else. Some of the kids might tease you about your height. Ignore the teasing and try to focus on the benefits of being tall—after all, you can reach high shelves and see through a crowd more easily!

I've heard that there is some kind of medicine you can take to get taller. Is this true?

A medication called growth hormone is occasionally prescribed by doctors for unusually short children whose body isn't producing a normal amount of growth hormone. Growth hormone is the chemical in the body that promotes growth.

The treatment with growth hormone is given in shots over a period of time. It doesn't necessarily make these kids taller than they would be otherwise (unless given in high doses). But growth hormone gives them a better chance to reach their potential height. If you have more questions about growth hormone treatment, talk to your doctor.

I heard on the news that it's important to build strong bones when you're a kid. Why?

Building strong bones at this time in your life will help you avoid potential problems like weakened bones later in life. A healthy diet—especially getting enough calcium—is the most important thing you can do to keep your bones (and teeth) healthy and strong. *Calcium* is a mineral that enables your bones to grow strong. You can find calcium in dairy foods like milk, cheese, and yogurt, and in some vegetables like broccoli and greens. Calcium is also added to other foods, such as some orange juices and tofu.

Exercise also plays an important role in keeping your bones strong—another reason to get lots of physical activity throughout the week!

Why does my doctor test me for scoliosis? What is scoliosis, anyway?

The spine of a person with *scoliosis* curves to the left or to the right instead of being straight. Scoliosis usually develops during the years when children are going through their growth spurt, sometime between the ages of 10 and 16.

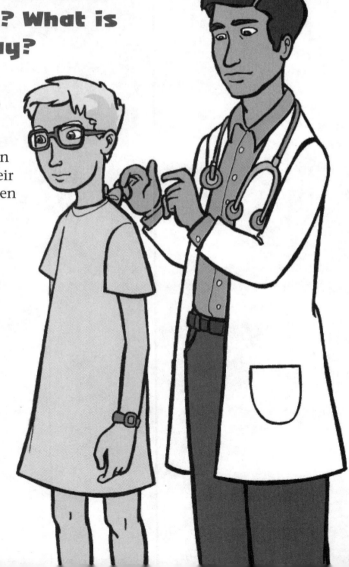

If the curve is mild, it doesn't require any treatment. If the curve is significant, the doctor may recommend special exercises to help straighten it. Sometimes surgery or other treatment is necessary to correct the curve.

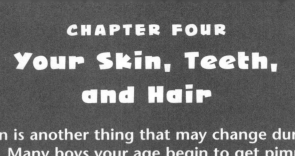

CHAPTER FOUR
Your Skin, Teeth, and Hair

Your skin is another thing that may change during puberty. Many boys your age begin to get pimples. Although pimples can be annoying, they usually go away over time, so don't spend too much time worrying about them.

Another change you'll notice is growing hair in new places on your body. Many boys are excited about getting facial hair and may even look forward to growing a mustache, a goatee, or a beard. Growing facial hair can make boys feel they really are growing older!

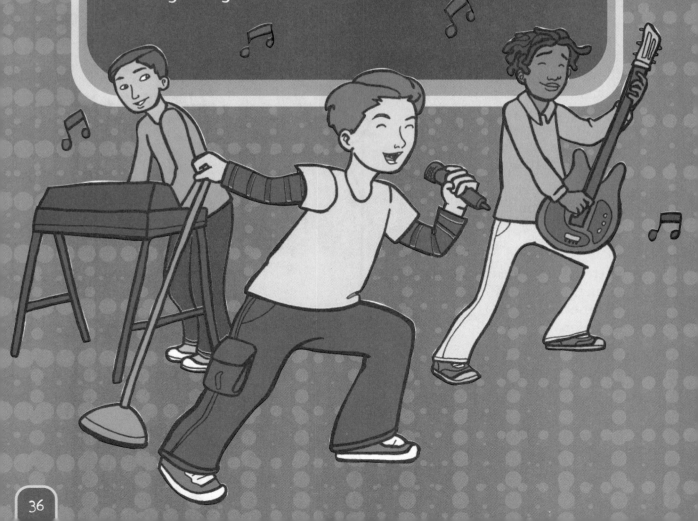

Why do I have pimples all of a sudden?

During puberty, your body begins to produce more hormones, like the male hormone testosterone. Hormones are chemicals that control many processes in the body. Male hormones, or *androgens*, can also increase oil production by the skin.

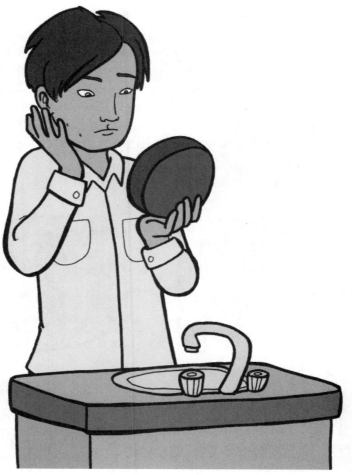

A mixture of oil and skin debris, called *sebum*, can sometimes get trapped in the *hair follicles* (openings in the skin through which hair grows). Then, if *bacteria* get into the blocked follicle and multiply, they can cause a reaction (called *inflammation*) that creates a *pimple*. (Bacteria are always present on your skin and usually cause no problems.) Pimples are filled with a substance called *pus*, which is produced when your body tries to fight the bacteria inside the blocked follicle.

Can stress affect my skin?

Yes, being stressed out or very worried about something can cause pimples. You may notice that your skin breaks out at stressful times, like before a big test, an important game, or a talk you have to give in class.

What are blackheads and whiteheads?

Blackheads, which look black on the surface of the skin, are blockages of sebum in hair follicles that have turned dark because they're exposed to oxygen in the air. *Whiteheads*, which look white on the surface of the skin, are follicles that are filled with the same material as blackheads but they have only a tiny opening in the skin. Whiteheads are white because the air can't reach them through this tiny opening. If the sebum inside the hair follicle can't get out and it builds up along with the bacteria, the blackhead or whitehead can turn into a pimple.

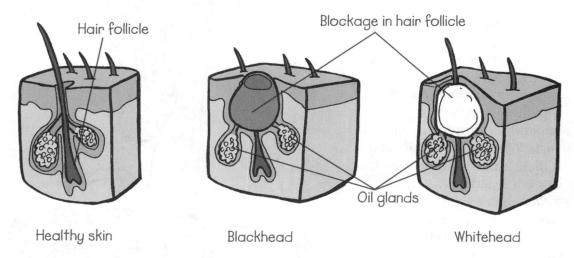

Hair follicle

Blockage in hair follicle

Oil glands

Healthy skin   Blackhead   Whitehead

What is acne?

If you have several blackheads, whiteheads, and pimples, you have *acne*. Although acne usually develops on the face, it can also occur on the neck, back, chest, buttocks, and, sometimes, the upper arms and thighs. Acne usually clears up in the late teens, although some people get it later in life. Sometimes, taking certain kinds of medications, such as corticosteroids, can cause acne. If you have acne after you start taking a medication, talk to your doctor.

How do I get rid of my pimples?

Whatever you do, don't pick at your pimples. Squeezing, poking, or pushing at a pimple can irritate your skin and make the pimple worse. Picking pimples can cause permanent scars.

You should keep your skin clean, but don't over-clean it! Too much scrubbing or scraping will irritate your skin and make your acne worse. Instead, wash your face twice a day with a mild soap. Drugstores have many products that can help with pimples; ask your doctor to recommend one. He or she will probably suggest a product that contains *benzoyl peroxide* or *salicylic acid*. (But *don't* use benzoyl peroxide and salicylic acid products at the same time because it could irritate your skin.)

You'll notice that these products come in different strengths. The doctor will probably recommend starting with a lower strength. Apply it to your skin once or twice a day. Your skin may seem to get worse at first, but that is normal. If your skin gets irritated, try using the product every other day or every third day. (Be careful when using benzoyl peroxide because it can stain your clothes.)

If after a few weeks your skin doesn't look better, see your doctor. He or she may give you a prescription for a different acne medication, may prescribe an *antibiotic* to help your skin (by fighting the bacteria), or may recommend that you see a dermatologist. A *dermatologist* is a doctor who treats skin problems. There are many effective medications available for treating even severe acne.

What other kinds of skin conditions could I get?

You may notice other skin conditions besides acne as you begin puberty. If you notice anything new or unusual, including signs of the skin conditions described below, see your doctor. He or she will identify the condition and tell you how best to treat it.

◆ **Warts**   Lumps with a rough surface that are caused by a virus. (Viruses are germs that can cause different kinds of infections, including the common cold.) Warts often develop on the wrists, fingernails, the backs of the hands, and the face. Some types of warts, called plantar warts, occur on the bottoms of the feet.

◆ **Moles**   Round or oval spots on the skin that are usually dark brown. Some moles are flat and some can be raised. If you have a mole that has looked the same for a long time but now has an irregular shape or is bleeding or sore, show your parents. They will probably want the doctor to look at it to make sure there's nothing to worry about.

◆ **Eczema**   Red, itchy patches on the skin that sometimes join together. The skin can become dry and lighter or darker than the surrounding skin, and, after too much scratching, may look like leather. Eczema often occurs on the inner part of the elbows or behind the knees.

◆ **Psoriasis**   Patches of thick, raised skin that are pink or red and covered with silverish white scales. It can occasionally cause mild itching or soreness. Psoriasis most often occurs on the knees, elbows, and scalp.

◆ **Acanthosis nigricans**   Raised, darkened patches on the back of the neck, armpits, or groin that make the skin look dirty. Occurs most often in young people who are very overweight and it is strongly linked to type 2 diabetes. Losing weight helps the patches disappear. If you think you have acanthosis nigricans, you may want to ask your doctor about it.

Did you know that your skin is actually your body's largest organ?

What else do I need to do to take care of my skin?

The obvious answer is to be sure to bathe or shower every day. In addition to producing more oil as you reach puberty, your body will also begin producing more sweat. And your sweat might begin to have an odor.

Most boys notice that they have odor, especially under their arms, around their penis and scrotum, and on their feet. Regular showers or baths—with soap and water—are the best defense against body odor. Also make sure you wear clean clothes, including clean socks, each day or after a workout and use deodorant and foot powder as needed.

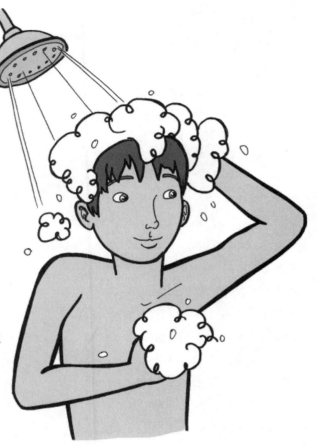

My parents are always telling me not to spend so much time in the sun and they always make me wear sunscreen. What's the big deal?

Too much exposure to the sun can be very harmful to your skin. A sunburn and a tan are signs of skin damage caused by the sun—that's how your skin protects itself. Over time, this skin damage can lead to skin cancer. Although rare, even young people can get skin cancer. Too much sun is also the major cause of wrinkles.

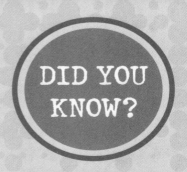

Use your sunscreen—save your skin!

There are many types of sunscreen from which to choose. The brand you choose is not important but the SPF is. *SPF* stands for "sun protection factor" and it's listed on the product label. The lowest, least-protective SPF you can find is 2; the highest is 50. Use a sunscreen with an SPF of at least 15 every time you plan to be outside. If you're very fair-skinned or tend to burn, use an SPF of 30 or higher.

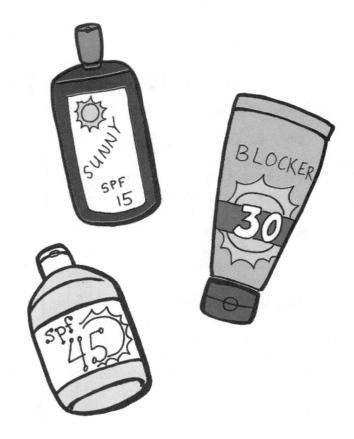

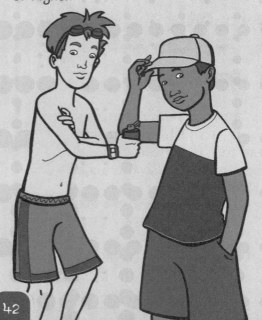

Your parents are right—you should wear sunscreen whenever you're outside. Don't forget to apply it to places on your body that get a lot of sun, like the tops of your ears, the back of your neck, and the tops of your shoulders. Try to limit the time you spend in the sun during the midday hours—between 10 a.m. and 3 p.m.—when the sun is most powerful and most dangerous. It's also a good idea to wear a cap, hat, or visor to help protect your head and face.

And stay away from tanning salons! Tanning in a machine can be just as bad for your skin as tanning from the sun.

What is jock itch?

Jock itch is an itchy, scaly rash caused by a fungus that occurs around the genital and groin areas. Many boys get jock itch. It's especially common among athletes who wear elastic shorts or jock straps, which tend to make the groin area warm and moist; the fungus is more likely to grow on moist, warm skin.

You can treat jock itch with an over-the-counter cream that you can get at a drugstore; ask your parents or doctor what medication to use. You apply the cream to the affected area. It also helps to keep the area clean and dry.

Lately, my feet sometimes smell. What can I do?

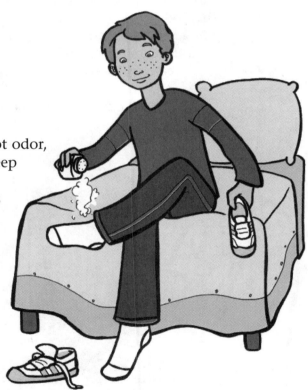

Like body odor, foot odor can be embarrassing. One way to avoid foot odor, or to keep it to a minimum, is to keep your feet as clean as possible at all times. Also wear cotton socks; socks absorb sweat from your feet. Avoid shoes that are made of plastic, rubber, or other man-made materials. These materials don't allow air to reach your feet, causing your feet to sweat and, possibly, smell.

If your shoes smell, buy an over-the-counter foot powder product. Powders that target food odor by absorbing sweat are available at most drugstores. Most are easy to use—you just sprinkle the powder onto your feet and into your shoes. If the odor remains, you could have an infection called athlete's foot; check with your doctor.

Hey! Never try to give yourself or a friend a piercing, and never let a friend give you a piercing. This can result in a serious infection.

Are piercings and tattoos safe?

Some kinds of piercings can be safe. For example, it's usually perfectly safe to get an ear pierced by a professional. Sometimes you can find a doctor who is willing to pierce your ear (or ears) in his or her office. Do not pierce your ears yourself or have a friend do it.

Even when done by a professional, body piercings can get infected, especially in parts of the body other than the ears (although piercings in the upper ear along the hard, curved part can sometimes cause hard-to-treat infections). It may be trendy to have a pierced tongue, but it can get infected and swollen—making eating, speaking, and even breathing difficult. A tongue piercing can also cause gum disease and can damage or chip your teeth.

Some piercings are very painful and can take a long time to heal. For example, navel and nipple piercings can take up to 5 months to heal—or longer than that if they get infected. Piercings in some parts of the body are more likely to get infected repeatedly. Sometimes you can take a piercing out and the hole may never fully heal, leading to a permanent scar. These are all things to consider before you decide to get a piercing.

Tattoos are also risky and can cause infections. Unlike most piercings, tattoos are permanent. It's very difficult—and expensive—to have a tattoo removed, and it can leave scars. Remember that you may like the idea of a tattoo now, but that doesn't mean you always will.

Both body piercings and tattoos can cause overgrowths of scar tissue called *keloids*. Boys who have dark skin are especially prone to forming keloids. If you tend to form keloids, you probably don't want to damage your skin in any way, with either a piercing or a tattoo.

If you still decide to have a piercing or get a tattoo, run your plan by your parents and a doctor before you do anything. Then make sure you carefully follow any instructions you are given for taking care of the piercing or tattoo to avoid infection and help it heal properly.

Most states regulate places that provide tattoos and piercings to ensure that they are safe. Currently it is against the law in most states to provide a tattoo to anyone under age 18 without the consent of a parent. Many states make it illegal to provide a body piercing to anyone under 18 even with a parent's consent. You do NOT want to get a tattoo or body piercing from a place that is not regulated—it's unsafe and against the law.

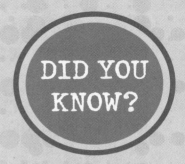

DID YOU KNOW?

Temporary Tattoos

Why not experiment with temporary tattoos? They're much safer and a great way to express yourself. You can be creative and change your art whenever you get tired of a tattoo!

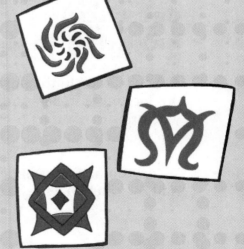

Why do I have to brush and floss my teeth every day?

You may not realize it now, but healthy teeth and gums are very important for your whole body's health. If you allow bacteria and other germs to grow in your teeth and gums, your teeth can decay and you could lose them. These germs can also make your gums bleed and your breath smell bad.

But most harmful to your health, the bacteria in your mouth can go to other places in your body and cause serious problems, even with your heart. That's why your parents are always reminding you to brush your teeth every morning and night, and sometimes more often (for example, if you have braces). Listen to your parents—and see the dentist every 6 months for a checkup and cleaning to make sure your teeth and gums stay healthy.

When will I start to grow underarm hair?

There is no exact answer to this question. The hair under your arms can begin to grow at almost any time during puberty. It usually happens after you have already started growing pubic hair (at pubic hair stage 4; see page 48).

Does having hair under my arms have anything to do with using deodorant?

As you learned in the previous chapter, certain parts of the body tend to produce more sweat—and more odor—during puberty. You have glands under your arms that attract bacteria. These bacteria, when combined with sweat, can cause an odor.

When you have hair under your arms, the sweat may feel stickier than it used to. And the smell may stay in your underarm hair.

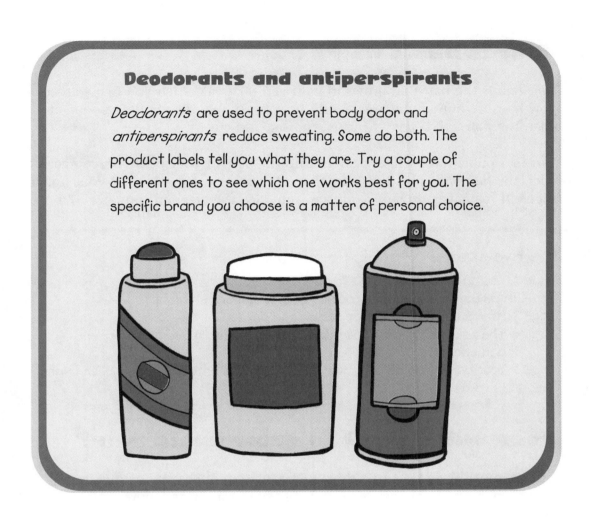

Deodorants and antiperspirants

Deodorants are used to prevent body odor and *antiperspirants* reduce sweating. Some do both. The product labels tell you what they are. Try a couple of different ones to see which one works best for you. The specific brand you choose is a matter of personal choice.

In addition to bathing, showering, and wearing clean clothes every day, using a deodorant or an antiperspirant can also help prevent or reduce body odor. It can also make your sweat feel less sticky.

Some deodorants can be sprayed on, some come in liquids that are rolled on, and some come in a gel or stick. If you have a skin reaction like a rash after using a deodorant, it could be because it contains aluminum. Some people are allergic to aluminum. Try a product that doesn't contain aluminum.

What is pubic hair?

Pubic hair is the hair that grows in your genital area. When you first start to grow hair in your genital area, it will be soft, thin, and straight. As you get older, the hair will become thicker, coarser, and curlier.

Your first pubic hairs will appear around the base of your penis. As you get older, the hair will spread up over the pubic bone and down onto your upper thighs. It may also grow on your scrotum. (See the diagrams on page 57.)

The five stages of pubic hair growth:

Stage 1: You do not have any pubic hair yet.

Stage 2: You begin to see a few pubic hairs, which are straight.

Stage 3: Your pubic hair becomes curlier and darker.

Stage 4: The hair grows over the pubic bone and usually becomes thicker and coarser.

Stage 5: Your pubic hair gets thicker and grows out onto the upper, inner thighs.

When will I start to grow pubic hair?

You will most likely start to grow pubic hair soon after you begin going through puberty. Pubic hair will probably start appearing before you develop hair on other parts of your body, like your underarms and face. But, just like everything else that happens during puberty, this can happen at any time. Some boys grow pubic hair earlier or later than other boys.

When will I start to grow facial hair?

Most boys start to see hair growing on their face sometime between the ages of 14 and 16. Your facial hair will develop after you have gone through a few other stages of puberty, including the growth of pubic hair, the penis, and the testicles.

Where will I first notice facial hair?

You will probably see your first facial hairs on your upper lip area, near the corners of your mouth. At first, these hairs will be soft, and they probably won't be very dark. Over time, these hairs will become darker and thicker. They will also start to cover the entire area above your upper lip. If you let them grow, you'll have a mustache.

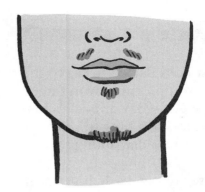

Next you will notice hairs growing on your cheeks and down from your sideburn area. You may also grow some hair below your lower lip. The last hairs to grow will be on your chin. If you let your chin hair grow in fully, you'll have a beard.

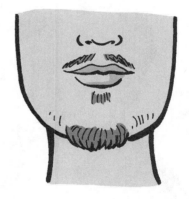

Not all boys will be able to grow a full beard. How much hair you have depends somewhat on heredity. Look at the men in your family and notice how thick the hair on their face is; this can give you an idea of what you can expect.

You may not finish developing facial hair until you're in your 20s. Not having a lot of facial hair now does not mean that you won't have more when you're older.

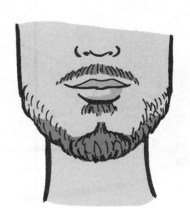

How do I shave?

Most boys decide to shave their facial hair. You probably won't need to shave every day at first. When you want to learn how to shave, ask your dad or an older sibling to show you.

Never share razors with anyone else because of the risk of infection.

There are two basic types of razors: disposable and electric. Electric razors are less likely to cause cuts but they don't shave as closely as those with blades. There are two types of disposable razors. One type is used a few times and the entire razor is thrown away. The other, more expensive and sturdier type has a razor head that you change but keep the handle. You'll notice that razors have different numbers of blades. A good choice is one that has double or triple blades that allow you to get a closer shave.

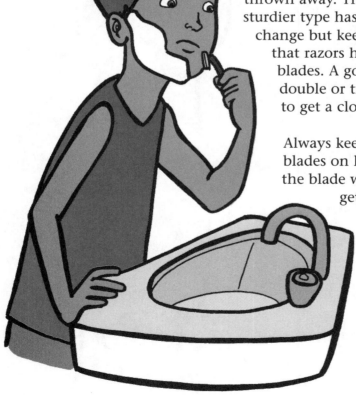

Always keep a supply of new razors or blades on hand. You'll need to change the blade whenever you notice it's getting dull. If you shave every day, you might change blades once every week or two.

How do you shave with a disposable razor?

Here are the basic steps for shaving with a disposable razor:

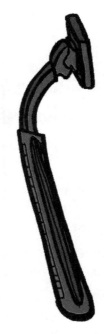

- Wet your face thoroughly with warm water. This softens up your facial hairs in preparation for shaving.

- Spread some shaving cream onto your face, which helps soften the hair even more.

- Press the blade gently against your skin and move the razor downward.

- After each stroke or two, rinse your blade with warm water to keep it from getting clogged with hair and shaving cream.

- Start with your cheeks and then move to your upper lip; leave the chin for last because the hairs there are toughest.

- Rinse off the blade when you're finished.

- Use your hands or a washcloth to rinse your face. Wipe off any remaining shaving cream and check to make sure you haven't missed any hairs.

- Pat your face dry with a towel.

- Apply moisturizer to your face to keep your skin from getting irritated. But make sure the moisturizer is *non-comedogenic* (check the label), so it doesn't promote pimples.

Always shave in the direction your hair grows to avoid shaving bumps, also known as *folliculitis*. And don't forget to change the blade frequently. If you don't, the blade will become dull and is more likely to cause shaving bumps and cuts.

How do you shave with an electric razor?

Here are the basics for using an electric razor:

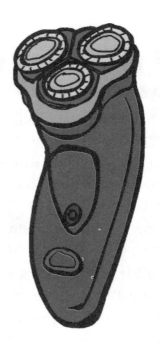

- Make sure your face is dry. Do not wet it before shaving with an electric razor.

- Move the razor gently over your face—you don't need to press it into your skin.

- Keep the razor clean by following the directions that came with it.

What should I do if I develop a skin problem from shaving?

If you notice that your skin has gotten really irritated with red bumps or an itchy rash, you have a skin condition called folliculitis. If your facial hair is very curly, you are more prone to getting folliculitis from shaving. This is because very curly hair is more likely than straight hair to grow back into the skin after shaving, causing ingrown hairs and irritation.

Acne medications that contain benzoyl peroxide, which you can find at most drugstores, can help relieve the rash. If this doesn't clear up the rash or if it gets worse, see your doctor. It could be infected and you may need an antibiotic to clear it up.

When will I start to grow chest hair?

Chest hair tends to develop much later in puberty. It's unusual for younger teens to have any chest hair. How much chest hair you will eventually have is largely determined by heredity. Once again, look at the men in your family to get an idea of how much hair you'll have as you get older and where it might grow.

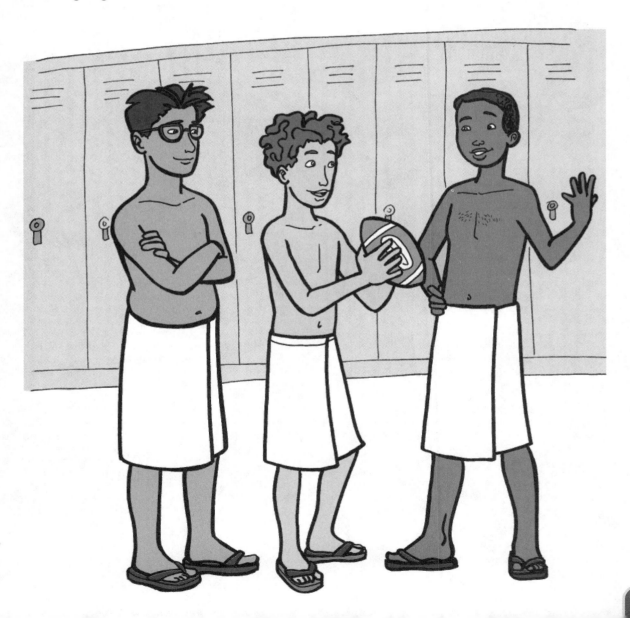

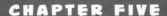

CHAPTER FIVE
Your Reproductive System— Inside and Out

Most boys are curious about how their body, especially their *genitals,* will change during puberty. Is what they see normal? What might not be normal? But many boys don't know who to ask or don't feel comfortable talking to anyone about it. You should know that you're not alone: Boys are often curious about these changes. This chapter will answer many of the most common questions boys your age have.

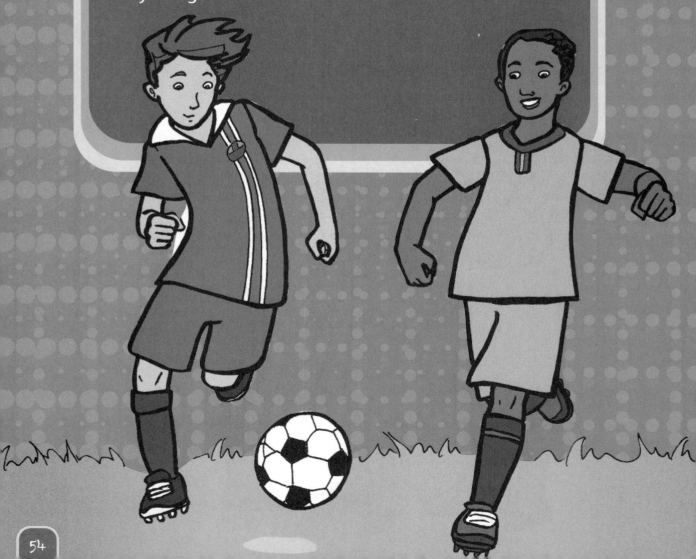

What *are* the testicles and the scrotum, actually?

The *scrotum* is the skin sac below the penis. Inside the scrotum are two *testicles* suspended by the *spermatic cords* (more about spermatic cords on page 56). The testicles produce the male hormone *testosterone* and *sperm cells*. (When a sperm cell from a male fertilizes an egg cell from a female, pregnancy can take place.) The scrotum is designed to protect the testicles. You may notice that one of your testicles hangs lower than the other; don't worry about this because it's normal.

> *Testosterone* is the major male sex hormone. Testosterone is responsible for sperm production and it gives you male characteristics such as facial hair.

To be able to make sperm, the testicles need to be in a special, protected environment. They need to be at a slightly colder temperature than body temperature—that's why the scrotum hangs outside your body. You will notice that sometimes your scrotum pulls in closer to your body and sometimes it seems to hang lower. When you're cold, your scrotum pulls in close to your body to keep the sperm warmer. When you're hot, it pulls away from your body so the sperm cells don't get too warm.

What is the penis made of?

Your *penis* is made of soft, spongy tissue that has lots of blood vessels. The dome-shaped head of the penis is called the *glans*. The rest of the penis is called the *shaft*.

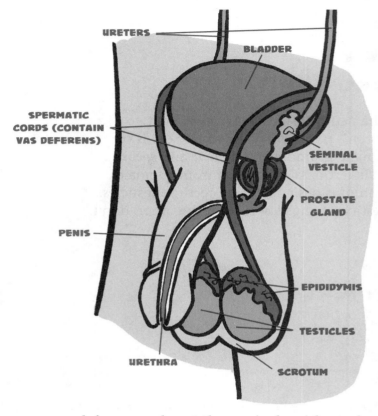

URETERS

BLADDER

SPERMATIC CORDS (CONTAIN VAS DEFERENS)

SEMINAL VESTICLE

PROSTATE GLAND

PENIS

EPIDIDYMIS

TESTICLES

URETHRA

SCROTUM

What reproductive organs are inside my body, and what do they do?

A number of *organs* inside your body handle sperm production and transportation. Inside the scrotum, each testicle is suspended by a *spermatic cord*, which contains blood vessels, nerves, and a tube called the *vas deferens*. On top of each testicle is a small storage area for sperm as they leave the testicle; this storage area is called an *epididymis*.

Before ejaculation (when sperm leave the body), sperm travel from the epididymis through the vas deferens and past the *seminal vesicles* and *prostate gland*. The seminal vesicles and the prostate gland produce a fluid that mixes with the sperm; this fluid is called *semen*. During ejaculation, semen exits your body through the *urethra*, the tube inside the penis that also carries urine out of your body. (For more details about ejaculation, see page 66.)

Why does my penis get hard sometimes?

Most of the time, your penis is soft; this is called being *flaccid*. When a boy is feeling sexual (and sometimes even when he isn't), blood rushes into the penis, filling most of the blood vessels and tissue and making the penis larger and harder. This is called an *erection*.

When an erection ends, much of the blood leaves the penis and goes back into the body. The penis then returns to its normal soft state.

My penis curves to one side. Is this normal?

It's normal to have a penis that curves slightly in one direction. Everyone's penis looks different. If you're worried about the shape of your penis, talk to your doctor. He or she will give you a medical evaluation and help reassure you that your penis is normal. Do not try to change the shape of your penis or bend it back because this could be dangerous.

How will my genitals change as I get older?

Your testicles will grow as the first sign of puberty, before your penis starts to grow. This moves you to stage 2 of puberty. This is also a sign that you are about to start your growth spurt in height.

During stages 3 and 4, the testicles and scrotum will continue to grow. The penis gets slightly longer but not much wider during stage 3. (Most boys reach stage 3 between ages 10 and 14.) The penis gets wider as well as longer during stage 4. (Many boys reach stage 4 around age 13 or 14, while others don't reach it until they're 17.)

Stage 4 is also the time when height increases the fastest.

In stage 5, your body will finish developing and you will reach your adult size. Many boys reach this stage between the ages of 14 and 16, but other boys reach it later.

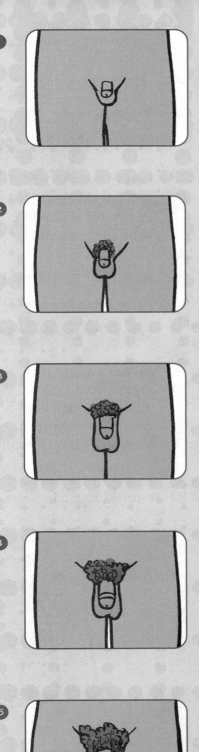

I worry that my penis is too small. How do I know if I'm normal?

Lots of boys worry about the size of their penis. It's important to know that size has nothing to do with how your penis functions. Penises vary slightly in size from boy to boy. And if you are at an earlier stage of puberty than your friends and classmates, your penis will probably be smaller for a while.

What's the difference between a circumcised penis and an uncircumcised one?

All boys are born with a fold of skin that covers the head of the penis (the glans). This skin is called the *foreskin*. *Circumcision* (removal of the foreskin) may be done in the hospital in the first day or two after birth. Some religious groups have practiced circumcision for thousands of years and continue to have their boys circumcised, sometimes in a religious ceremony.

A circumcised penis looks different from a penis that hasn't been circumcised but it doesn't in any way affect how the penis functions.

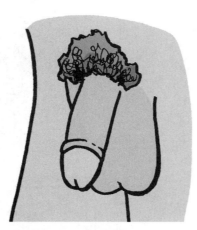

Circumcised penis

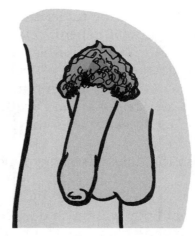

Uncircumcised penis

What should I know if I'm not circumcised?

If you are uncircumcised, you have skin, called the foreskin, that covers the head of your penis. This skin can be pulled back to reveal the head of the penis. When you pull back the foreskin, it's called retracting it. The foreskin also retracts naturally during an erection.

When you're young, it can sometimes be difficult for the foreskin to retract. But over time, it will separate completely from the head of the penis and retraction will be easier. Don't worry if you notice that your foreskin does not fully retract. If you're experiencing any pain, however, talk to your doctor about it. You should *never* force the foreskin to retract.

Some boys occasionally notice that their penis is sore and swollen and they can't pull back the foreskin. This could be a condition called *phimosis*, which can occur when the foreskin gets stuck to the head of the penis. If you think you could be having this problem, see your doctor immediately. If it's not causing symptoms, it doesn't need treatment and you will probably outgrow it. Sometimes treatment with medicated creams can help. But if you continue to have pain and swelling and have difficulty urinating, the doctor may recommend a surgical procedure such as a circumcision.

How should I take care of an uncircumcised penis?

If you are uncircumcised, be sure to always keep the area under the foreskin completely clean. All you need to do is pull back your foreskin while you shower and thoroughly clean the head of the penis, especially where it meets the shaft of the penis.

If you don't clean it regularly, a substance called *smegma* can build up under the foreskin. Smegma has a strong, unpleasant odor. This condition can be avoided with careful and thorough washing.

Why do I need to worry about cancer in a testicle? I'm only a teenager.

Testicular cancer is one of the most common *cancers* in males between the ages of 15 and 35. This is why you need to know about it and check yourself regularly, especially once you turn 15. Check your testicles about once a month so you become familiar with their look and feel and can easily find anything new or unusual.

The best time to do a testicle self-exam is during a shower or after a warm bath. Here's how:

◆ Using both hands, place your thumbs on top of one of your testicles and your index and middle fingers under the testicle.

◆ Roll the testicle gently between your thumb and fingers for about 30 to 60 seconds to feel the entire surface of the testicle.

◆ Feel the surface of the testicle for any lump or swelling.

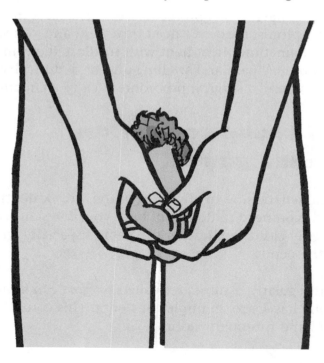

- Repeat the above steps with the other testicle.

- Stand in front of the mirror and check your testicles and scrotum for any swelling or to see if one testicle seems noticeably larger than the other. (It's normal for one testicle to be slightly larger than the other.)

- If you notice any lumps or swelling in your testicles, see your doctor right away.

I have some light-colored bumps around the head of my penis. Is something wrong?

These bumps, which tend to grow in rows around the head of the penis, are called *pink pearly papules*. They are harmless. They seem to occur more frequently in uncircumcised males.

You do not need any treatment for pink pearly papules. But when you are sexually active, have them checked out by the doctor to make sure that's what you have. When you are sexually active, bumps or marks on your penis could come from a sexually transmitted disease (STD). STDs require quick treatment because they can lead to serious problems when not treated. When in doubt, always ask your doctor.

If you notice anything new or unusual about your penis or testicles, don't be shy about telling one of your parents or your doctor. You want to make sure there's nothing to worry about.

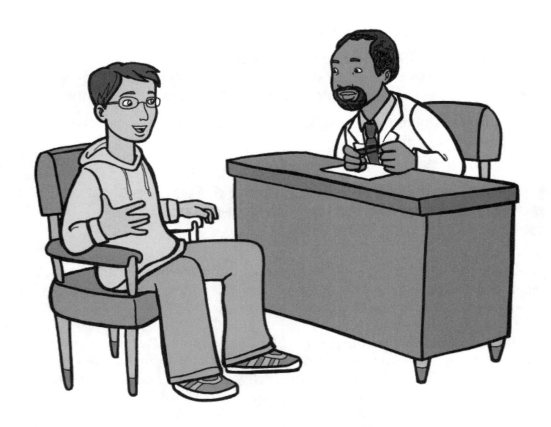

I felt something soft and bumpy in my scrotum. What could it be?

You should definitely visit your doctor if you feel anything unusual in your scrotum. It could be something like a *varicocele*, a harmless condition in which the veins in the scrotum become wider and stretched and may feel like a sack of worms when you touch them. Varicoceles usually develop on the left side and occur in as many as 15 percent of teenagers.

Or you could have a *hydrocele*, which is a buildup of fluid around the testicles. Or you could have a *hernia*, which occurs when part of the intestines bulges into the scrotum or into the groin area. Hernias and hydroceles are less common than varicoceles in adolescents.

It is always important to check with your doctor right away if you have any pain in your genitals, if you have a sudden change in your genital area (such as a new hydrocele or varicocele), or if you notice anything else different. Most problems are easy to treat when taken care of quickly.

My doctor says I have undescended testicles. What does that mean?

Before a baby boy is born, his testicles are located inside his abdomen and then, before birth, they move into the scrotum. Sometimes, however, a boy is born with one or both testicles still in the abdomen. This condition will usually be corrected by doctors while the child is still very young. Rarely, a boy still has an undescended testicle by the time he reaches puberty. Talk to your doctor if you are worried that you may have an undescended testicle.

I have lumps under my nipples and they sometimes feel sore. What's happening? Could I be growing breasts?

Up to half of all boys notice these lumps under one or both nipples during puberty, usually between ages 10 and 14. This is caused by the changes in hormones that can occur at this time. In almost all cases, this is not a cause for concern and your chest will return to normal within about 18 months. Still, for reassurance, it's a good idea to talk to your doctor about it at your next visit so he or she can follow-up with you.

CHAPTER SIX
Erections, Wet Dreams, and Masturbation

The previous chapter answered some questions you might have about your penis and other reproductive organs. This chapter addresses even more personal questions, like "Why do I get erections?" or "What is masturbation and is it okay to do it?" Use this chapter as a tool for learning. Also use it to realize that your questions and experiences are common and normal—it's perfectly okay and, in fact, important to think, talk, and read about these issues.

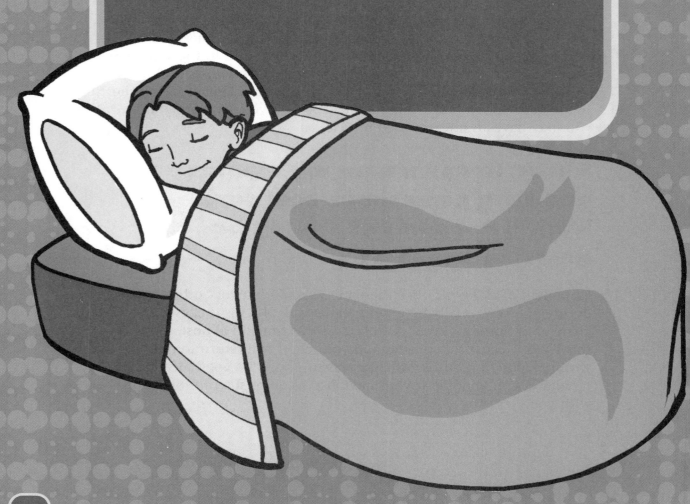

Why do I get erections?

Boys get erections when their penis is touched or rubbed. They also can get an erection when they're feeling excited, nervous, or sexual. Erections may occur when you're thinking or reading about something sexy, watching something sexy in a movie, or looking at something that excites you.

You may notice that you have an erection when you wake up in the morning. This type of erection is usually not caused by a sexual feeling. It can happen when you have a full bladder, which can affect some nerves in the penis and cause an increase in blood flow into the penis.

You may also get what is called a spontaneous erection, which seems to come out of nowhere. Many boys report getting an erection in the middle of class, even when they aren't thinking about anything sexual. As you begin puberty, you may notice that you get erections at odd times. This can be pretty embarrassing—especially because you can feel that you have no control over it! But this is completely normal. As you grow older, you will be better able to control your erections and these random erections will occur less frequently.

What do I do when I get an erection in an embarrassing situation, like in class?

An erection is very obvious to you, but that doesn't mean it's noticeable to anyone else. Some boys wear clothes like long shirts that cover their genital area in order to hide unexpected erections. Other boys use books or magazines to hide sudden erections. Another trick is to try to focus on something else. Clear your mind! Give it something else to think about.

Random erections usually go away quickly, so just try to relax and know that within a short time it will go away.

What is ejaculation?

Ejaculation is the process by which a thick, sticky, white liquid called semen leaves the body through the penis. You might remember learning in chapter 6 about how sperm are combined with fluids to produce semen. Let's review this a little to help explain ejaculation. It can also be helpful to refer to the drawing on page 56 to see the different parts of the reproductive system that are involved in ejaculation.

Your testicles are constantly producing new sperm. When you become sexually excited, your testicles and some other parts (like the epididymis, seminal vesicles, and prostate gland) have muscle contractions. These contractions cause sperm to leave the testicles through the epididymis and travel past the seminal vesicles and prostate toward the urethra. Muscle contractions in the seminal vesicles and prostate push out the fluid that combines with the sperm to make semen.

The final stage of ejaculation occurs when strong muscle contractions stimulated by strong sexual feelings push the semen through the urethra and out of the head of the penis. Ejaculation is also called *orgasm*. It may seem like a lot of semen comes out, but it's usually only about a teaspoon. If you haven't ejaculated in awhile it may be more or, if you've ejaculated recently, it may be less.

When will I ejaculate for the first time?

Boys ejaculate for the first time after their body has started to produce sperm. This usually happens sometime between the ages of 11 and 15 and coincides with the many other physical changes your body is going through. Like any other stage in puberty, some boys will be younger and some will be older when they first ejaculate. Some boys experience ejaculation for the first time by masturbating. Other boys ejaculate for the first time while they are sleeping (see the next question).

Sometimes I wake up with sticky pajamas. What happened?

Most boys ejaculate sometimes in their sleep. When this happens, it's called a *nocturnal emission*, more commonly known as a *wet dream*. While you're sleeping, you may have a sexual dream and ejaculate in your sleep. You probably won't remember the dream in the morning, but you know that something happened because your pajamas or sheets are wet and sticky. Wet dreams are a normal, natural body process and there is nothing you can do to prevent them. As you get older, you will have them less frequently.

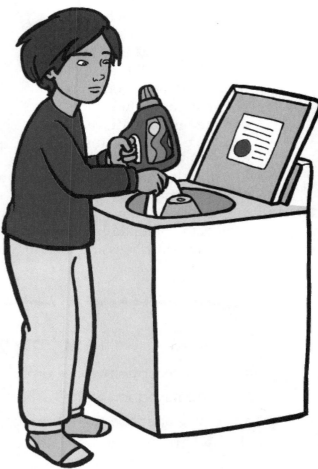

I hear some kids talking about blue balls. What's that?

"Blue balls" is a slang term for the pain that you might feel in your testicles when you have an erection for a period of time and don't ejaculate. This feeling is only temporary and the pain will go away by itself if you wait awhile. You can also choose to masturbate to relieve the feeling.

This discomfort is not a reason to try to get someone to do something sexual with you. The pain or discomfort is not a cause for concern and it will not in any way harm you, your testicles, or your ability to be sexual.

What is masturbation?

Masturbation is touching or rubbing the penis to feel good sexually. Most boys masturbate until they ejaculate (have an orgasm). You've probably heard lots of slang terms for masturbation and some of them can sound pretty silly. The fact that there are so many slang terms for masturbation shows you how very common it is.

For teenagers, masturbation is a safe way to relieve sexual tension without having to worry about pregnancy, having a sexual relationship with another person, or getting a sexually transmitted disease.

Masturbation is a normal, healthy way to explore your sexual feelings, express the natural sexual response, and safely experiment with sexual touching. Most boys and men masturbate, as do most girls and women.

MYTHBUSTERS

- Masturbation cannot affect your athletic ability or your vision.
- Masturbation cannot affect your looks.
- Masturbation cannot affect your ability to be sexual with a partner in the future.
- You do not run out of sperm no matter how frequently you masturbate because your body is constantly making sperm.

Can masturbating do anything bad to me? Is it possible to masturbate too much?

The answer is "no" to both of those questions. Again: Masturbation is a healthy, natural thing to do in private. It doesn't matter whether you masturbate once a month, once a week, or several times a day.

The only reason masturbation might be a problem is if you are choosing to masturbate so much that you don't have time for other things, like spending time with your friends or enjoying your hobbies. Otherwise, the amount you are masturbating is normal for you.

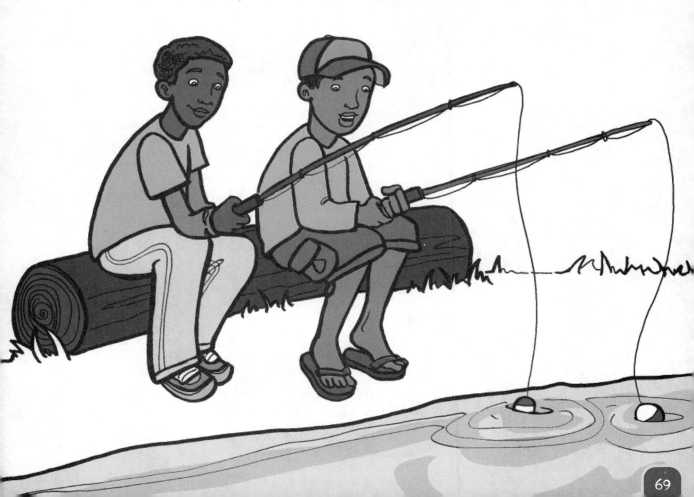

CHAPTER SEVEN
Your Feelings

This chapter is one that some boys may be tempted to skip. Why? Some boys don't feel comfortable discussing their feelings. Society sometimes sends out the message that it is not okay for boys or men to talk about their feelings. Boys and men are supposed to show strength and confidence.

Of course strength and confidence are good qualities to have, but it is also normal for boys to have times when they feel sad, stressed, angry, and lonely, and to show these feelings. Having feelings and being able to talk about them actually shows someone has a lot of strength and confidence. This chapter talks about the kinds of feelings that can sometimes be hard for boys to recognize and accept.

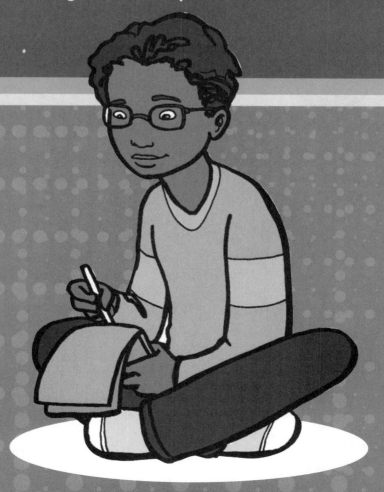

Why do my feelings seem to be changing so much lately?

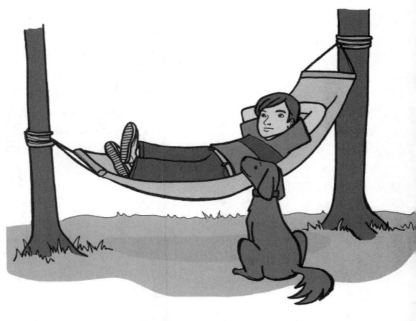

Depending on the day, the time, and the situation, a person can feel different from one moment to the next. Sometimes you may feel happy, other times sad, and other times stressed out. When you become a teenager, you may notice that your mood seems to shift more often than it did when you were younger. You might feel happy one minute, and then you suddenly find yourself feeling angry over something that's not that important.

Your body produces more chemicals called hormones during puberty. Hormones help control many body processes, including mood. As a result, your mood may shift more now than it did before. Also consider that you are probably going through many other changes in your life. You may have started middle school, your friendships might be changing, and you may not feel quite as connected to your parents as you used to. You may be starting to wonder about dating, and you may develop crushes. All of these things can make your life seem more complicated, and they can affect the way you feel.

I sometimes feel bad about myself. Why?

Many boys start feeling less confident during puberty. You may compare yourself more to others. You may worry that you are shorter, taller, fatter, skinnier, less muscular, or more developed than other boys in your classes. You may worry that you are not as smart, not as funny, not as athletic, or not as artistic as other people. Although these worries are normal, they can affect your self-esteem, how good you feel about yourself.

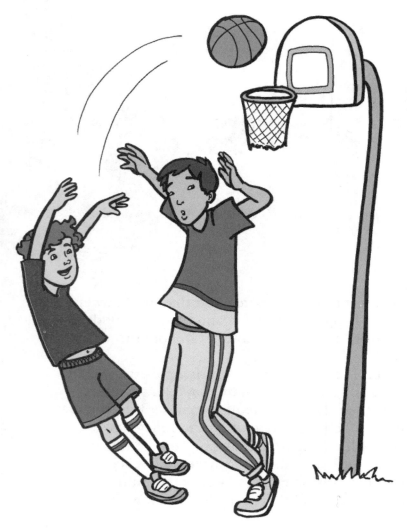

What can I do to feel better about myself?

What you think about yourself has a big impact on your self-esteem. Beware of negative self-talk. Examples of negative self-talk are "I'm the worst math student in this class" or "I'm never going to make the basketball team because I'm so short."

In order to feel better about yourself, find ways to turn your negative thoughts into more positive ones. You may have to practice this at first, just like any other skill you are trying to learn. It may feel a little silly when you start, but if you keep doing it, you will find that it helps.

Examples of positive self-talk might include: "If I study a little harder, I know I can ace that test next week." or "Many shorter guys are really good at basketball and, if I keep practicing, there's no reason I won't be good enough to join the team."

If you have been trying for a while to feel more positive and it is not working, talk to someone, like your parents, a favorite school counselor or teacher, or your doctor or other trusted adult.

It sometimes seems that my parents don't understand me anymore. Why?

Many boys notice that their relationship with their parents changes during puberty. You may be feeling that you are ready to be treated more like an adult. You may want to be allowed to make more decisions for yourself, and you may want more freedom. You may feel that you should be allowed to decide your own curfew, what you do after school, and where you go and what you do on weekends.

Your parents may not feel the same way. They may think you're not yet ready to make all of these decisions. As a result, you may be disagreeing more with them about these issues.

You may also discover that you are not interested in sharing as much information with your parents as you used to. When you were younger, you may have looked forward to coming home from school and telling your parents all about your day. Now that you are a teenager, you may not want to tell them quite as much about what's going on in your life. Parents who are used to knowing a lot more about their kids' lives might start asking them for more information. This can also sometimes lead to conflicts.

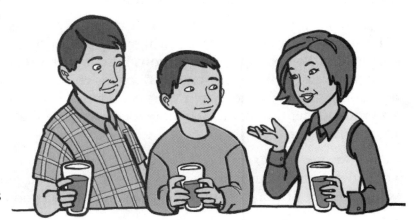

Although it is normal for teenagers to have some differences with their parents, try your best to figure out new ways to communicate. Read the tips on the next page to learn how.

How can I get my parents to listen to me?

Good communication requires some effort on both sides. How you approach your parents can make a big difference. If you have an important subject to discuss with your parents, it is important for you both to listen to each other. Here are some tips for improving the two-way communication between you and your parents. They also work well when chatting with people other than your parents!

- **Plan ahead** Find a time and a place when you can really spend some time discussing an issue you are concerned about—for example, when you and a parent are out for lunch or dinner, relaxing at home, or on a long car ride. (Sitting in the car outside school in the morning as the bell is ringing is *not* a good time for an important discussion.)

- **Prioritize** Figure out which issues are most important. If what you are hoping to achieve is some extra time with your friends after school, don't bring up other requests at the same time. Save those for another time.

- **Negotiate** If you are working on getting more privileges and freedom, you can increase your chances by showing your parents that you are more responsible. For example, take responsibility for getting all of your homework done without having to be reminded, or for chores like cleaning your room and doing your laundry. When your parents see you acting more grown-up and independent, they may be more likely to agree that you are ready for more privileges.

- **Compromise** For example, if you want freedom to spend more time with your friends and your parents are willing to allow you more time on the weekends but not on school nights, this might be a good compromise.

- **Take turns** Agree that both of you will take turns listening and talking. Neither of you can get your point across when you're talking at the same time. Practice the 5-second rule with your parents: You each wait 5 seconds before responding to the other.

What should I do when I'm feeling angry?

Anger is a normal feeling—one that *everyone* experiences from time to time. You might be angry after an argument with a friend or because you worked hard at something and it did not turn out the way you wanted. *Feeling* angry is fine. It's what you *do* with your anger that's important.

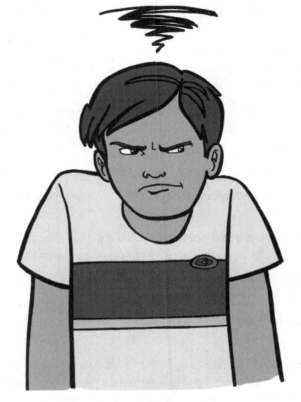

Although everyone feels angry sometimes, people handle their anger in different ways. Do you hold all your anger inside? Does it sometimes build up to the point where you explode? Or do you keep it hidden, to the point where it is all you can think about? Do you let your anger out right away, without thinking or worrying about who it affects? None of these are good ways to handle anger.

If you *don't* deal with your anger, it can affect you in many negative ways. Holding angry feelings inside can even make you physically sick—for example, you might begin to notice that you are getting headaches or stomachaches. If you let your anger out in an aggressive way, you may find that you have hurt yourself or someone else. Learning how to deal with your anger now will definitely make your life easier later.

If you are having difficulty managing your anger, you might find these tips helpful:

◆ Talk about your feelings using "I" statements. Start with "I feel angry because…." Don't accuse the other person of doing something wrong. Instead, focus on *your* feelings.

◆ Talk about what would help make you feel better. Try something like "I would feel less angry if we didn't always have to compete."

Sometimes it is best to cool off before you talk directly with the person who made you feel angry. Here are some tips to help you calm down:

◆ **Do something physical.**   Go for a long walk or run, ride your bike, or skateboard.

◆ **Write down your feelings.**   It doesn't have to be perfect writing. Just get those angry feelings out. They're safer on paper than exploding at a friend!

◆ **Do something relaxing.**   Listen to your favorite CD, play a computer game, or watch a movie.

◆ **Let your feelings out.**   Punch a pillow, find someone to talk to, or cry. Yes, cry—every boy needs to cry once in a while.

If you're still finding it hard to overcome your angry feelings, talk to someone. Once again, a parent, a school counselor, or another trusted adult, can help you figure out more positive ways to cope with your anger.

I wish I felt more comfortable around people. What can I do about being shy?

Many boys struggle with feeling shy during puberty. Feeling shy can be tough because it can make you not want to try new things, participate in school activities, or go to social events like school dances or parties.

These tips might help you overcome your shyness:

◆ **Be patient with yourself.**   Learning how to be more outgoing can be hard work—but that doesn't mean you *can't* do it!

◆ **Start small.**   Try talking to a couple of people in the hallway. Say "hello," ask a quick question, or offer some help with a school project. Slowly work your way up to inviting a new person to do something fun, like coming over to your house to play video games or shoot baskets.

◆ **Join a group.** Participating in a group such as a club or team gives you the opportunity to meet new people who have the same interests as you.

Some of these tips might seem hard at first, but with time and practice they *will* get easier to do. Try to remember that no one knows how you feel inside. You may be feeling terribly nervous, but if you keep a smile on your face and a friendly tone in your voice, others will see you only as friendly.

Lately I've been feeling stressed out. What can I do about it?

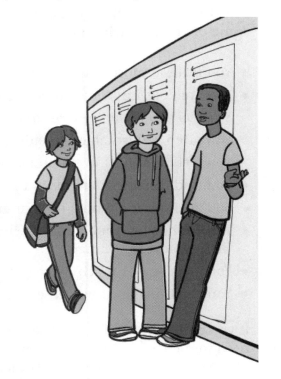

Most kids say that they are more stressed during their teenage years than they were when they were younger. You probably have more homework, harder classes, more responsibilities at home, and more disagreements with friends or parents. No wonder you feel stressed! Although a certain amount of stress is normal, too much of it can be harmful to your health. Make an effort to set aside time in your busy schedule to do things you like. Play your musical instrument, go for a bike ride or swimming, finish your woodworking project, or exercise or work out. Do something every day that you enjoy and that makes you feel good. Make sure that you're taking good care of yourself. You need to get enough sleep and to eat healthy foods. Also, it is important to limit how much sugar and caffeine you eat or drink. Lack of sleep and a bad diet can make you feel even more stressed out.

If your stress level is *really* high, talk to someone. Let your parents, your doctor, or another trusted adult know what's going on.

Sometimes I feel really unhappy. Should I be worried?

Everyone experiences sadness once in awhile. It's normal to feel down when you are struggling with school work or when you lose a good friend or don't make a team you tried out for. These bad feelings usually pass pretty quickly and you start to feel better.

But if you notice that you are not feeling better and you are dealing with some of the following symptoms, you may be experiencing depression:

- You feel sad most of the time and are crying more often.
- You aren't as interested in your favorite activities.
- You feel bad about yourself most of the time.
- You often feel irritable, sometimes toward friends.
- You feel tired most of the time.
- You find it harder than usual to concentrate.
- You are skipping school or your grades are going down.
- You are having trouble eating enough or you're eating more than usual, even when you're not hungry.
- You are sleeping much more or much less than usual.
- You can't imagine you will ever feel better.

If you *ever* feel like hurting yourself or feel that life is not worth living, you need immediate help! Tell your parents or another trusted adult as soon as you can. No one should have to feel that down. There are things that can be done to help you start feeling better.

If a friend ever shares with you that he or she is thinking of hurting himself or herself, *do not* keep that information secret. Your friend needs help, *immediately*, so tell someone right away! Talk to your parents or another trusted adult and let them know what is going on. It may feel like you're betraying a friend, but you may actually be saving his or her life.

My grandfather recently died and I'm confused about what I'm feeling.

You may be feeling grief. Grief is a strong feeling of sadness that people experience when someone close to them dies. You can also experience grief at other times, such as when you lose your best friend, your parents get divorced, or a pet dies. You may be feeling sad, hopeless, lonely, scared, confused, or guilty—or all of those at different times.

It helps to talk about your feelings with other family members who are also experiencing the loss. It can also help to talk with other people who have lost a loved one. You will realize that you are not alone—other people have similar feelings.

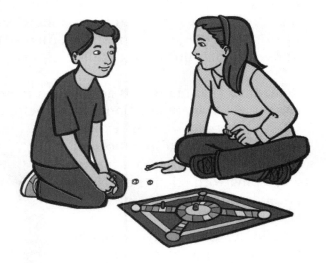

Everyone experiences grief in his or her own way but most people tend to follow a common pattern. At first, many people have a feeling of numbness because they are having a hard time accepting the death and they may even deny it for awhile. They may feel alone, empty, and in shock during this first stage of grief. Then, they may begin to feel guilty and angry, and they may even take their anger out on the people who are closest to them. In the next stage, people usually experience intense feelings of sadness and loneliness. After a time, these intense feelings begin to calm down and they start to gradually return to their normal routine.

The final stage of grief is when you are able to accept the death or other loss and begin to enjoy your friends and activities again. You will still think about your grandfather, but with less pain. Eventually, you will be able to remember him with happiness.

I recently found out that my parents are separating. What can I do?

When parents separate, divorce, begin dating new people, or get remarried, it's natural for their children to feel upset. In these situations, it's normal for kids to experience strong emotions. If you are experiencing changes like these at home, you may feel angry, scared, lonely, confused, or even guilty. You may feel powerless or that your life is on hold, or resentful at having to go back and forth between two homes. As hard as it may seem, it's important at this time to take care of yourself. Continue to follow your dreams, participate in your favorite activities, spend time with friends, eat right, and be physically active. Those are the things you can control, and they'll help you feel better, too.

Remember that many kids go through these situations—you are not alone. It can help to talk to other kids who are experiencing similar things. It's also important to talk to your parents about how you are coping with all of these changes and how they are affecting you.

> **Hang in there! Things may feel very tough right now. But try to remember that your parents don't love *you* any less just because *they* are separating.**

You do not always have to put on a brave face—your parents don't expect you to be strong all the time. They know that sometimes you may need to cry, yell, or just talk it out. Also, it is important for kids to speak up because their parents may be so caught up in work and other activities that they sometimes may not recognize their teen's feelings.

If you find that your feelings are becoming overwhelming, that your grades are slipping, or that you are having trouble sleeping, you need to let your parents, your doctor, or another trusted adult know. You deserve to, and can, get help dealing with these difficult changes in your life

I feel weird talking about my feelings.

Many boys find it hard to learn how to talk about their feelings. It can sometimes feel strange, embarrassing, or awkward. The truth is that everyone needs to talk about their feelings. Reaching out to others for support is actually a sign of strength—*not* weakness. You'll be surprised at how much better you feel, and you will find that everyone has these same feelings from time to time.

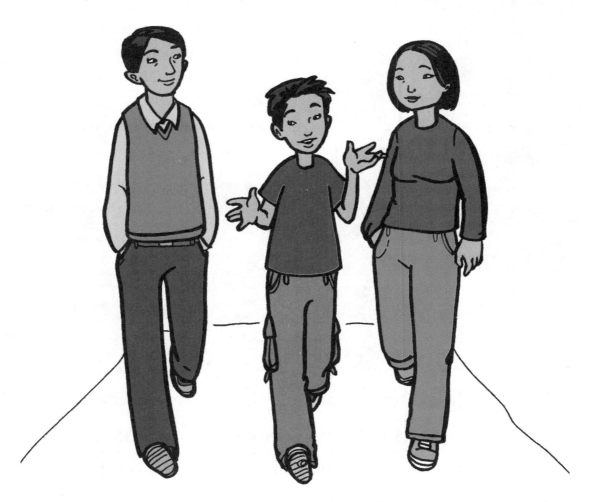

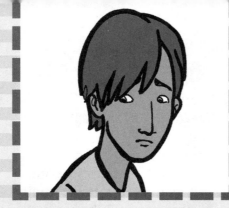

REAL BOYS, REAL FEELINGS

I like this girl in my class but she doesn't know I'm alive. I try to think of ways to get her attention. I think I'm just going to talk to her after lunch. Age 12

My parents separated in September and I worry they'll get divorced. I want them to stay together but I don't know how to get them to. Age 13

My friend and I want to see a PG-13 movie. My friend told his parents that it was OK with my parents, but it didn't work. His mom called my mom and my mom told her I'm not allowed to see PG-13 movies either. Age 13

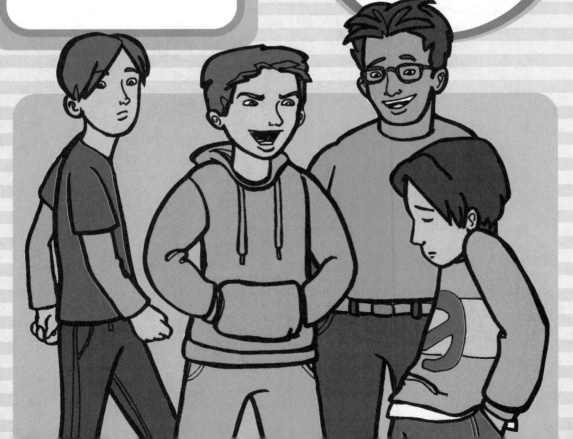

My mom and dad decided they were going to live in different houses. Now I live with my mom and see my dad on weekends. I hate it because I want to live together again. Age 11

One of my friends called me a wimp because I cried in school. Now, I'm scared to show my feelings. Age 12

I used to be popular but now I feel kinda stupid a lot of the time. I spend more time alone than before. Age 11

CHAPTER EIGHT
Relationships

One of the most important parts of your life now is just being with your friends. Whether it's going to the movies, shooting baskets, or just hanging out at a buddy's house, being with your friends is a top priority. This chapter will help you learn how to form healthy relationships—both how to find good friends and how to be a good friend.

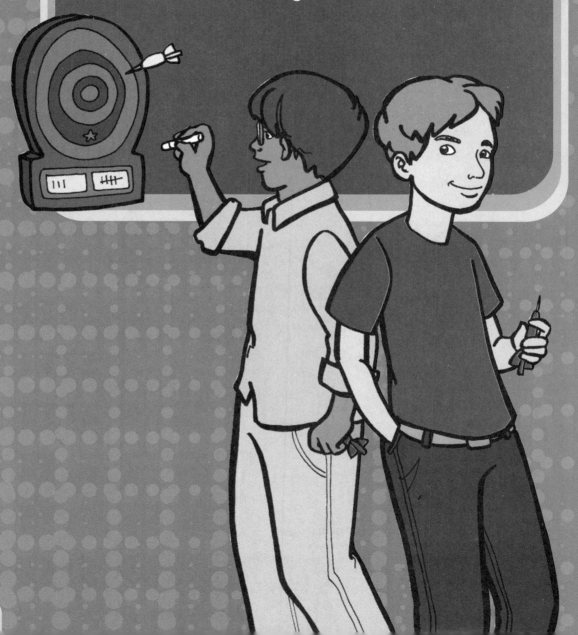

What makes a good friend?

Different boys might have different answers to this question. But most would agree on the following qualities.

A good friend...

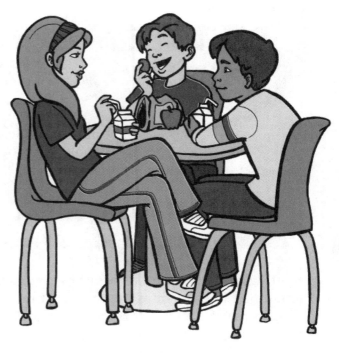

... is someone you can count on.
... is someone you can trust.
... is considerate of your feelings.
... listens when you need to talk.
... makes you feel good about yourself.
... likes some or many of the same things you do.
... may have some differences from you but it doesn't affect your relationship.

How do I make new friends?

When you become a teenager or start middle school, you may find that you want to make new friends. You may be the kind of boy who finds making friends easy—you are outgoing and it's no big deal for you to walk up to someone new and start a conversation. If this does not sound like you, however, making new friends might seem harder.

One way to make new friends is to find an activity you enjoy in which you might also meet new people. For example, if you enjoy music, try out for the school band. If you like sports, join a local team. If you are into art, find a local art center and join a group. Or just sit next to someone new at lunch or offer a bag of chips to someone to start a conversation.

How do I keep a good friend?

Good friends are important. Sure, they're great to have around for the fun times. But they can also help you feel better when times are tough.

In order to keep a good friend you need to be a good friend. Look back at the list of qualities on page 85. Do you have those qualities? What do you expect from your friends? Are you as supportive of them as you'd like them to be of you?

Many boys say that what they care about most in a friend is that he or she is trustworthy. If you make sure that you are there for your friends, chances are they will do the same for you.

What should I do when I'm arguing with a friend?

Most fights between friends start over something small that builds into something bigger. For example, a fight might start when a friend teases you about a new haircut. At first the teasing might seem funny, but then you may start feeling annoyed and even embarrassed—especially if it's happening in front of other people. Then you might start making fun of your friend in return, saying things like "Oh yeah, you think my haircut is lame? Well at least I don't have such bad teeth!" Before you know it, this war of words has escalated either to the point where you and your friend have a physical fight or to the point where you can no longer stand to be around each other.

Many boys communicate with each other by "playing around." In other words, they spend much of their time together teasing each other. This can be okay if it doesn't happen too much and the teasing doesn't get too personal or mean. But since it can often turn into an argument, it might be better just to avoid teasing friends all together. At the very least, it's important to know when to stop; be aware of clues that you may have gone too far, such as if your friend looks down or turns away from you or even avoids you.

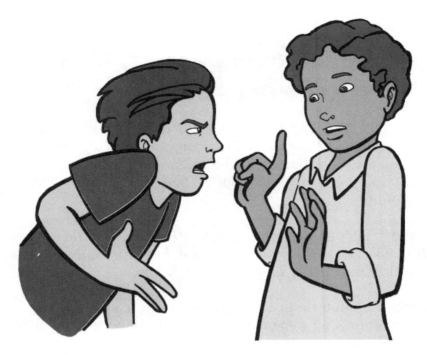

What do I do if an argument is about to turn physical?

Sometimes when people get really angry at each other it might feel like the only solution is to start hitting each other. Still, physical fighting will never solve anything—as you have probably already learned. If you have a physical fight with a friend, it can be incredibly hard to ever fix the friendship. Plus, you both may end up hurting each other.

Sometimes boys experience pressure to get into physical fights. You may hear things like "Why aren't you fighting him? You're such a wimp!" It can actually take more courage to avoid a fight than it does to let yourself be pressured into one. By not letting another person urge you into a fight, you are making your own decision—not allowing others to decide your actions. Be confident and just walk away—you will be the "bigger" person and others will realize it too. If you feel that a situation is escalating to the point where a physical fight might happen, it's okay to ask for help. Let your parents or another trusted adult such as a teacher or counselor know what's going on.

What happens if my good friend and I are growing apart?

This will happen a lot as you get older and your interests change. You might notice that you don't have as much in common with a friend as you used to. Still, you don't want to hurt someone's feelings in this situation. It can be hard to talk about growing apart, but it's better to talk it over than to just drop your old friend.

If you notice that a friend seems to be putting some distance in your friendship, it's okay to ask what's going on. Sometimes people don't realize how what they're doing is affecting other people.

But sometimes friends do just grow apart. If this happens to you, concentrate on making some new friends or work on improving other friendships you have.

We're in middle school, but one of my friends acts like he's still in elementary school!

Do you remember reading back in the beginning of the book about how boys go through puberty at different rates? Well, some boys are ready to act more grown-up before other boys are. You may be into "teen stuff" like parties, you may be dating, or you may like different kinds of movies and books now. Or you may still be into some of the familiar games and toys you've liked for the past couple of years. Either way is completely normal.

It can be hard, though, when friends are interested in very different things at different times. Sometimes these friendships stay strong because, deep down, the two friends still have a lot in common. Other times the friendship does not seem to work anymore. It's okay to grow apart, as long as no one does anything to hurt the other person in the process.

What is a clique?

A *clique* is a group of friends that behaves exclusively—that is, it excludes, or leaves out, other people. Cliques tend to develop in middle school. Friends in cliques may dress alike and they often have the same taste in music, sports, or other activities. They stick close together, making it hard for newcomers to join the group.

Many kids feel left out of cliques. Kids who are not in cliques sometimes feel they don't fit well into any of the groups in their school. Sometimes kids who are in cliques feel bad, too, because they feel they must always act a certain way.

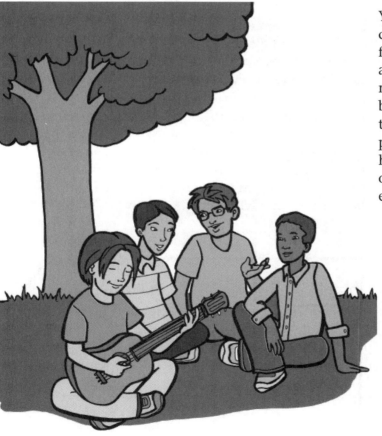

You may be in a clique, or you may feel the need to be in a clique, but keep in mind that cliques can be very limiting. And they will definitely prevent you from having a wider variety of friends and experiences.

I keep hearing about peer pressure. What is it?

People who are your age, like your classmates, are called your *peers*. Because you spend so much time with your peers, you naturally learn from each other. When you influence each other to do something, it's called *peer pressure*. Peer pressure can be either positive or negative.

Positive peer pressure is when someone influences you in a positive, constructive way, like studying hard, being kind to older people, helping out at home, and avoiding alcohol and drugs. Positive peer pressure is a good thing.

Negative peer pressure is when someone tries to get you to do something you know is not healthy or smart, like cheating on a test, drinking alcohol, cutting class, lying to your parents, or shoplifting. This pressure may come in the form of bribes, dares, nagging, or even threats.

Even if other kids are not obviously trying to get you to do something, you may give in to peer pressure on your own to, say, smoke cigarettes, because you want to be accepted by the group or "fit in." Or maybe you're afraid that the kids in the group will make fun of you if you don't go along. It's important to learn how to resist giving in to peer pressure that can be harmful. The next couple of questions will give you some ideas on how to make good choices.

It may not seem possible at your age, but the choices you make at this time in your life can have a lasting impact—both good and bad—on your future. So think hard before you act—and try to make good choices!

Some of my friends have started shoplifting. They keep asking me to do it with them but I don't want to. What should I do?

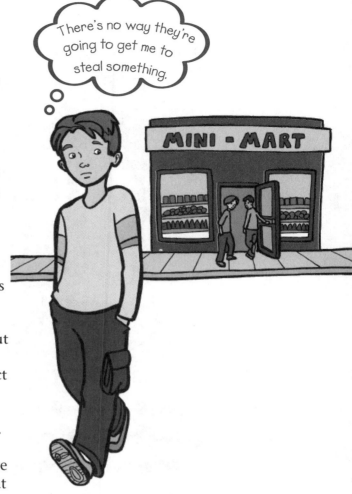

Deep down, you know that stealing is wrong and you don't want to get in trouble. You also don't want your parents to be disappointed in you. But keep in mind that the consequences of shoplifting can have a lasting effect on you—it's simply not worth it to allow yourself to be pressured into doing something you know is wrong.

Tell your friends there's no way you're going to risk getting into trouble, that your parents would be really mad and ground you for who knows how long. You can also suggest something else to do, or say you need to get home and you're already late. Or just simply walk away from the situation. Maybe you could "peer pressure" your friends into not shoplifting!

In the end, if your friends really care about you, they will respect that you need to make your own decisions. Also, good friends don't want their friends to get into trouble and should support them when they decide they don't want to do something they know is wrong. This group of kids may not be the best choice in friends. You may want to find friends who share your values and don't try to get you to do things you truly don't want to do. That way, everyone benefits!

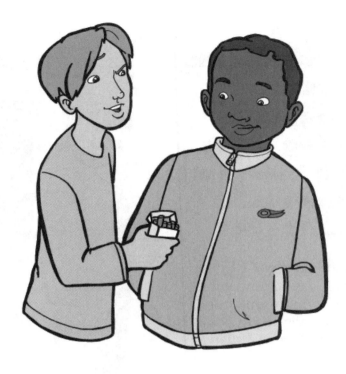

What should I do if my friends are trying to get me to try using drugs, alcohol, or cigarettes?

Everyone has heard the advice to "Just say no!" in response to pressure to do something you know is wrong. Your parents and your teachers have probably also talked to you about it. You always have the choice to say, "No, I don't want to do that" or "No, I don't feel like doing that" and walk away from something that could be harmful. This is always the wisest course. Go home, go to class, join a group of friends, or talk to someone else.

You can also tell your friends why you have made a decision not to try drinking, smoking, or using drugs. Be firm and confident as you explain your reasons. You can say that you know these substances are dangerous, that they can be physically addictive, and that they can interfere with school, family, and relationships and harm your health. Presenting your reasons will let your friends know that you have thought about it and that you are serious when you say "no." It might also help them make better decisions and choices. Saying "no" to peer pressure can also help you realize who your good friends are. Good friends will support your decisions and respect your feelings.

As a general rule, avoid situations where kids might be drinking or doing other risky things. For example, stay away from houses where the parents aren't home and kids are gathering for a "party." Also avoid parties where you know alcohol or drugs will be available. You can always use your parents as an excuse. It's as simple as saying, "I want to go to that party, but you know what my parents are like. They'll ground me for the rest of the year if I get caught." Your parents want you to use them as an excuse in these kinds of situations! They will be proud of you for figuring out ways to keep yourself out of possibly dangerous situations.

> In addition to saying "no" to your friends who are trying to get you to do things you know you shouldn't do, give your reasons for not doing them. Another good approach is to suggest other things to do such as: "Let's go to a movie." "Let's work on that project together." "Let's go play baseball."

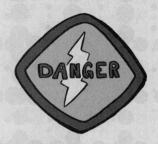

Inhalants

To get high, some kids are breathing in fumes from common household products like hair spray, cleaning fluids, and spray paint. Using inhalants, or "huffing," is extremely dangerous because these chemicals can make your heart beat irregularly and even make it stop—no matter how young you are. Inhalants can also cause sudden death from suffocating or from choking (usually on vomit). If you are using inhalants, stop now. If you can't stop using them, get help. Talk to your parents or another trusted adult right away. Your life could depend on it!

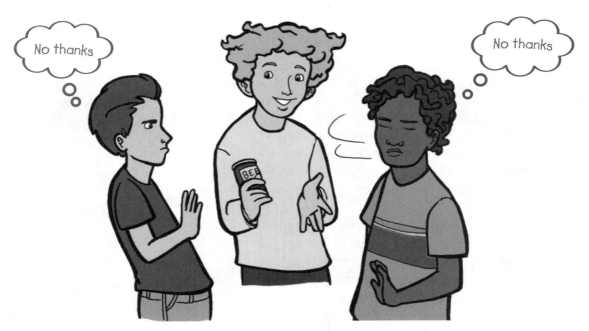

What if I'm thinking about trying drinking or smoking, like some of my friends?

You may be curious about alcohol and cigarettes because you think they are grown-up things to do, or you have heard stories from other kids about trying cigarettes or alcohol. Some of these stories might make these habits sound fun or exciting. The reality is that the younger you are when you start smoking or drinking, the more likely you are to become addicted and experience the negative effects of these habits on your health. Even at your age, these behaviors can harm your health. For example, smoking can affect your lungs and reduce your ability to excel in sports, drinking can make you more likely to engage in risky behavior such as unsafe sex or riding with a driver who has been drinking. An excess of alcohol can be fatal, and some drugs such as inhalants can cause sudden death.

> **People who drink beer and wine can become dependent on alcohol, just like people who drink hard liquor.**

If you are even thinking about trying smoking or drinking, talk to your parents or another trusted adult. It's important to think it through before acting and to get help understanding the safety issues involved. You could also do some research on your own about smoking or drinking. The Internet has lots of resources that will help you understand the dangers of these behaviors (see pages 112 to 115 for some good Web sites). Another option is to talk to a teacher or your school nurse. They will probably have lots of information to share about the risks of starting to smoke or drink when you're young.

What is bullying?

The broad definition of *bullying* is physically attacking, threatening, teasing, or purposely excluding someone to make him or her feel bad. When people think of bullying, they imagine a bigger kid pushing a younger kid around or forcing a younger kid to give up his lunch money or bicycle. This is an obvious type of bullying. But most bullying is less obvious than that.

Bullying is not just between kids who don't know each other very well. It can also happen between friends. For example, let's say you often sit on the school bus with the same group of boys. One day you get on the bus and the other boys are laughing at you and then ignore you when you sit down, making it obvious that they don't want to be with you. You feel terrible. You later find out that one of the boys has said something untrue about you to make everyone snub you. This can be an act of bullying. You can probably think of lots of examples of bullying you've seen at your school.

Marijuana— Just as harmful as cigarettes

Some people think that marijuana is not as harmful as cigarettes. But they are wrong. Smoking marijuana can have the same damaging effects on your lungs, heart, and blood vessels that smoking cigarettes does—including lung infections, lung cancer, heart disease, heart attack, and stroke. Also, heavy use of marijuana can produce a psychological dependence that can make you lose your energy, ambition, and motivation and have problems dealing with normal, everyday stress.

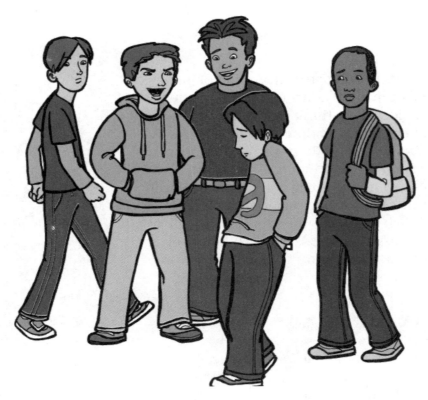

Another kind of bullying involves the Internet. It even has a name—*cyber bullying*. Some boys claim that other kids have posted false information or rumors about them online or sent an e-mail to someone pretending to be them. Kids are also using text messages on cell phones to bully other kids.

Sexual harassment, when someone makes unwanted sexual comments to a person or touches a person in a sexual way without his or her permission, is a form of bullying. To learn more about sexual harassment, see page 108.

What do I do if I am being bullied?

Bullying is never okay. And bullying is very hard to deal with all alone. If you are being bullied, tell your parents, some friends, teachers, a school counselor, or another trusted adult about it. You need all the support you can get when fighting a bully.

Some kids choose to try to ignore bullies. After all, bullies are basically trying to get attention so people can see how "important" they are. If you don't give them the attention they want, they may become frustrated and bored enough to give up trying to make you feel bad. But if that approach doesn't work, get other people involved to help you.

What do I do if a friend is being bullied?

If you have a friend who is being bullied, it's important to stand up for him or her. Let the person being bullied know that you are there to support him or her. If you see someone you don't know well being bullied, try to go over and help him or her walk away from the situation.

If one of your friends is being the bully, talk to him or her. Explain that you don't like what he or she is doing. Remember that bullies often pick on people because they are insecure. They believe—mistakenly, of course—that if they can make someone else feel bad other people will think they are a "big shot."

Is it possible that I am a bully?

Do you make fun of people? Have you purposely left other people out of groups or activities or spread rumors about other kids? If so, you have acted like a bully.

Before you act like a bully again, think hard about how you would feel if someone bullied you—or a sibling or a good friend. You would feel pretty terrible. If you really try to consider other people's feelings, you are likely to realize that you don't want to do this to anyone after all. You might also see that bullying someone else does not make you look strong and powerful—it makes you look small and weak.

If you are having a hard time stopping yourself from being a bully, you need to get help. Talk to someone. Start with your parents or a school counselor. They can help you learn positive ways to deal with your negative feelings and behaviors toward other kids and figure out ways to form healthier friendships. Best of all, once you do away with your bully personality, you are sure to feel much better about yourself!

CHAPTER NINE
What About Sex?

An important part of puberty is becoming interested in things having to do with dating and relationships. These issues can be complicated at times. And you may find that you have lots of questions but are not sure where to go for answers. Your parents and other trusted adults are a good place to start—they'll be able to help and guide you. This chapter can also give you some of the answers you're looking for.

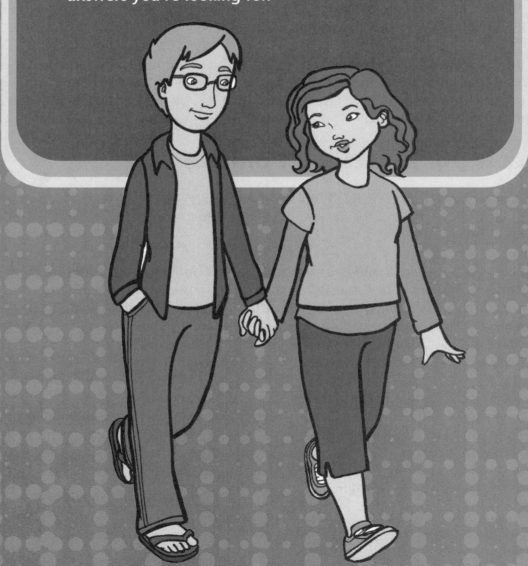

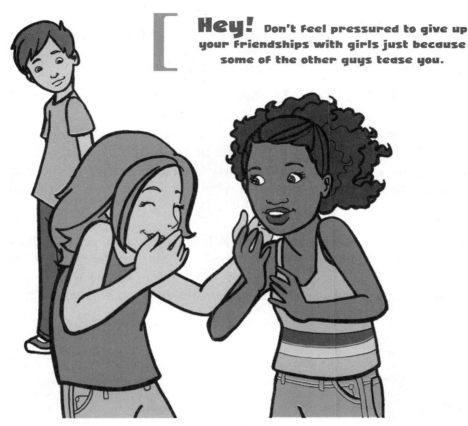

Hey! Don't feel pressured to give up your friendships with girls just because some of the other guys tease you.

Why does it seem that boys and girls suddenly don't have as much in common as they used to?

At your age, it may seem that you have less in common with the girls in your school than you used to. You may feel a little awkward around girls now because a part of you finds them really interesting and another part of you finds them kind of strange. Why are some girls giggling all the time, and what are they giggling about? Why do some girls act so grown-up?

You may not realize it now, but underneath it all you still have a lot in common with the girls around you. You're all going through similar things at school and you're all dealing with changes in your bodies. Also, you're all experiencing new emotions and changes in your way of thinking.

Why does it sometimes feel uncomfortable to be around girls now?

When you were younger, it wasn't a big deal to have a good friend who was a girl. But when you reach puberty, these friendships may seem a little more difficult. If you're spending a lot of time with a good friend who is a girl, other people might tease you about having a "crush" on her. You might also be teased if you like to hang out with a group of girls.

But it's important to have friendships with both boys *and* girls. If you limit your friendships to just boys, you are automatically eliminating half of the people out there who could very well be your good friends! You would also be limiting your experiences because boys and girls can sometimes have different views of things.

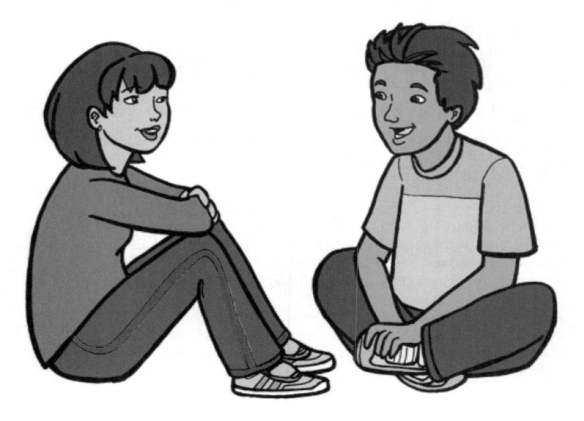

What, exactly, is a crush?

A crush is having romantic feelings toward someone. These feelings can build slowly over time or they can hit you suddenly. When you have a crush, you might find that you're thinking about your crush all the time. Or you might feel extra nervous when your crush is around, or you may even turn red or get sweaty palms when you're talking together. These are all normal responses to having a crush.

You can have a crush on almost anyone. You might have a crush on the person next to you in math class. Or you might have a crush on a teacher or on a character in your favorite TV show or movie. It all depends on who you find attractive.

What do I do if I have a crush on a girl?

You have a few choices. You can choose to keep your crush totally private and not tell anyone. Sometimes the feelings fade quickly, but other times it can take awhile.

You might choose to tell your friends about your crush and get their advice about what you should do. Be prepared, however, because they may want to get involved by telling your crush about how you feel. So tell them if this is what you do or do not want them to do!

Your final choice is to let your crush know about your feelings yourself. You might want to ask if she wants to have lunch together or if she would like to share your extra cookie. She may feel the same as you and will want to spend extra time together. Or you may sense that she does not have the same feelings. It's important to be ready for either possibility. If she doesn't feel the same way, you might just change the subject to something neutral, like "Did you get a ton of math homework today too?"

It can be very disappointing when your crush does not feel the same way you do, but remember that everyone has gone through this at some time or another. Your feelings, naturally, will be hurt at first. But you will probably soon develop a crush on someone else, and that will help you feel better.

What do I do if a girl has a crush on me?

If you like her, it can be exciting to let her know. But if you don't feel the same way, it's important to let her know in a nice way. The most important thing to remember is to always be respectful of other people's feelings. Treat her the way you would want to be treated in the same situation.

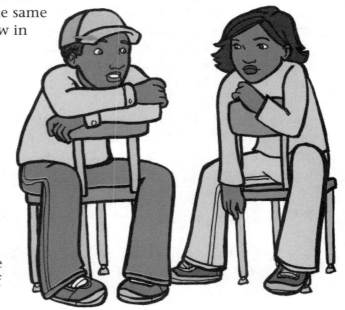

You could say something like "I'm sorry I don't feel the same way. But I really like you as a friend and I hope we can keep hanging out." You should also keep her feelings private. Imagine how embarrassed you would be if everyone knew you had a crush on someone who didn't feel the same way!

What if I have a crush on another boy?

It's not unusual for boys to have crushes on other boys. Having a crush on a boy does not mean you will not have crushes on girls. Figuring out who you are attracted to can be complicated. People can be attracted to different people at different times in their life.

You may find that you're only interested in boys, only interested in girls, or somewhere in between. If you feel confused or worried about these feelings, talk to your parents or another trusted adult. This person could be, for example, another member of your family, a school counselor, or your doctor. They can help you sort out your feelings.

When are teenagers ready to date?

There's no right answer to this question. First of all, you should check in with your parents to see how *they* feel about you dating. Some parents think it's okay for young teenagers to date, while others prefer that their kids wait until they're a little older. Some parents allow their kids to go on "group dates," in which several boys and girls go out together, but not on one-on-one dates.

You also need to ask yourself if *you* are ready to start dating. It's perfectly normal at your age to feel not yet ready to date. And, if you are *not* ready, you should not feel any pressure at all to start dating. Many young teens prefer to wait until they're older before they have to deal with a more complicated relationship.

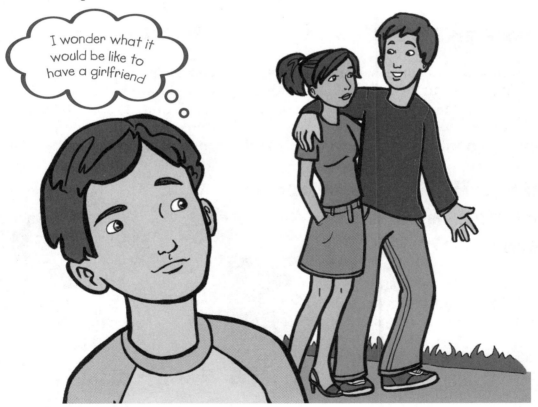

If you feel that your friends are giving you a hard time about not dating, it's probably because they are also feeling nervous about it. Stay confident in your ability to make the best decision for *you*, and encourage your friends to focus on their own decisions. In response to your friends, you might say something like the following:

◆ I don't feel ready to date yet.

◆ I don't want to date yet.

◆ I'm too busy with school activities.

◆ My parents won't allow me to date yet.

If you feel you *are* ready to begin dating, talk to your parents or another trusted adult. Dating can be very complicated, and having someone to talk to about it can be helpful.

How can I talk to my parents about dating?

This can be a hard conversation for many boys to have. You may be embarrassed about it and are afraid to even bring it up. But it is important to find out where your parents stand on this topic. So, take a deep breath and say something simple like "I think I want to start dating. What do you think?" Chances are, the conversation will get easier from there. See the communication tips on page 74.

How will I know when I'm ready to kiss someone?

Some of your friends may already have started kissing. But this does not necessarily mean that *you* are ready for it yet. Don't feel embarrassed if you're not ready—you will know when the time is right for you.

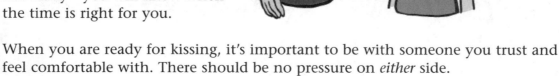

When you are ready for kissing, it's important to be with someone you trust and feel comfortable with. There should be no pressure on *either* side.

Sexual responsibility

Generally, kids who can talk openly with their parents and who have information about reproduction, sexuality, safe sex, and birth control are more likely to resist peer pressure and postpone having sex—or be responsible when they do have sex. Sexual responsibility means making decisions that respect each person's values and goals and increase self-esteem, not decisions that make anyone feel hurt, guilty, or ashamed.

Why is it better to wait until I'm older to think about being more sexual with someone?

There are many good reasons to wait until you are older to become sexually active. It is safer—both emotionally and physically—when you are older. There are lots of responsibilities involved in having sexual contact with another person, and it's important to wait until you feel ready to accept all of these responsibilities.

When you have *sex*, you have to consider the possibility of an unplanned pregnancy or getting a sexually transmitted disease (STD; see page 107). You need to know about birth-control methods that can prevent pregnancy, such as *condoms*. Condoms also reduce the risk of STDs. Bringing sex into a relationship can make the relationship a lot more complicated. There are many ways to feel close with someone without actually having sex. You can still be physically close with someone in ways that feel good but also keep you safe. Holding hands, hugging, kissing, and putting your arm around someone are all healthy ways to show affection.

What is sex?

There are different kinds of sexual activities. Two common ones are sexual intercourse and oral sex. *Sexual intercourse* is when the erect penis enters the vagina. *Oral sex* is when a person uses his or her mouth to stimulate another person's genitals. *Anal sex* is when the erect penis enters the *anus*. These are all sexual activities.

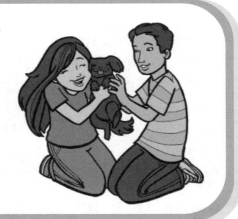

Some healthy ways to be close

- Walk together in the rain.
- Go to a friend's or a sibling's baseball game together.
- Play together with a new puppy.
- Go for a jog or exercise together.
- Watch a favorite movie together.

What should I do if my friends are pressuring me into having sex?

No one should pressure anyone into doing anything sexual. When you are ready to become sexual with another person, your decision will be based on your values—the things that you believe. Your values develop from your relationships with your family, your cultural or religious background, and your community. Your values may tell you that kids should wait until they're older before being sexual in any way. It is important to be true to your beliefs

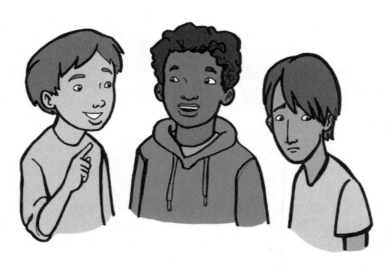

and not allow anyone to force you to go against them. After all, it's your body and your life—no one else's. Many kids who were pressured into having sex later wish that they had waited. It's important to respect your possible partner's decision as well. As always, these are good issues to discuss with a parent or other trusted adult.

Hey! Believe it or not, oral sex is really sex. You CAN get STDs, including HIV, from having oral sex.

What are STDs? How do people get them?

It is possible to get an infection called a *sexually transmitted disease* (STD) from having sexual intercourse, as well as from having oral sex or anal sex. Some STDs cannot be cured, some can make you unable to have children, and some STDs can lead to cancer. *HIV/AIDS* is an STD that can kill you.

Condoms are the only form of birth control that reduces the risk of infection with an STD. But keep in mind that condoms are not as good against some STDs as they are against others.

When you are ready to have sex, the best way to protect yourself is to *always* use a condom—each and every time, no matter what. If you don't have a condom or don't know how to use one properly, don't have sex! Sex using condoms is often referred to as "safe sex." In reality, however, it is only *safer* sex. The only 100-percent effective way to protect yourself from STDs is to not have sex. Some STDs don't cause any symptoms, so you might not realize you have one. If you think you might have symptoms, or you just want to talk more about the possible health effects of having sex, talk to your parents or another trusted adult, or make an appointment to see your doctor for more information and a health check-up.

MYTHBUSTERS

You CAN get a girl pregnant:

even if it's the first time you or she has had sex.

even if you have sex during her period.

even if you have sex standing up.

even if you withdraw your penis before ejaculating ("coming").

Behaviors that are never okay

Some forms of sexual behavior, such as those described below, are never okay and always need to be reported immediately and stopped.

Sexual harassment

Sexual harassment is when someone makes unwanted sexual comments to a person or touches a person in a sexual way without his or her permission. Sexual harassment is *never* acceptable. You have a right to go to school, play on a team, and live in a neighborhood without being harassed. And you should not harass others.

Both boys and girls report being sexually harassed in school. They have talked about being grabbed inappropriately in hallways and in locker rooms, or finding out that someone is spreading rumors about them that are sexual in nature.

If any of these things happens to you, tell someone immediately. Let your parents know. Tell a teacher or counselor, or go straight to the principal. Your school should take this issue very seriously and make sure that everyone can feel safe in the building.

Sexual assault

The law considers *any* unwanted sexual contact—even through clothing—to be *sexual assault*. If this ever happens to you, tell someone immediately. You should not feel embarrassed or ashamed. It is *never* your fault—you are *not* responsible for another's person's actions. Understand that you did not do *anything* to deserve the assault.

Some boys think that if their partners allow touching in a sexual way that they must continue to allow it. This is not true. If they want the touching stopped, or to go back to just being friends, boys must listen, respect their feelings, and not pressure them. If you pressure anyone into doing anything sexual, it is sexual assault.

Sexual abuse/molestation

Being touched in a sexual way by an older teen or an adult is *sexual abuse* or *molestation*—even if the person is a relative or friend. It is never okay for an adult to touch a child or a teenager in a sexual way. Sexual abuse is against the law. It is never the child's fault—even if the child "went along" with the touching. If you are sexually abused or molested, tell your parents or another trusted adult immediately. And keep telling until you find someone who will help. You have a right to feel safe.

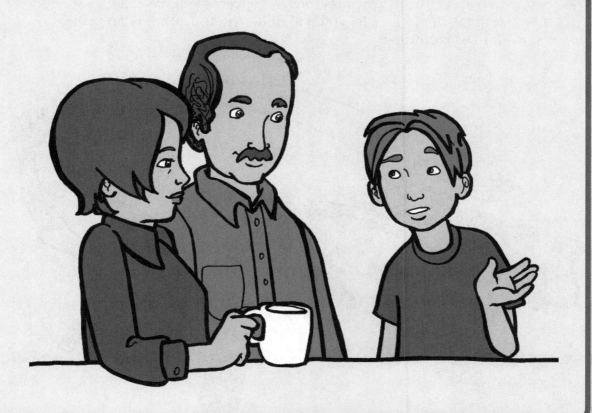

I still have a lot of questions about relationships. What should I do?

It's normal to feel confused and to have many questions about relationships during this time in your life. Reading about these issues is just one way to get some answers. Of course, you and your friends will probably talk a lot about all of these things. But it's also important to find trusted adults who can listen and give you advice.

How do you find adults who can help you and who you can trust? Good people to turn to first are, of course, your parents. Other people you can trust include doctors, nurses, teachers, coaches, school counselors, and grandparents, aunts, uncles, and other older relatives. They'll be happy to help you with any questions or concerns you have. Remember: If you keep talking to people, you will find, over time, that relationships seem a lot less confusing!

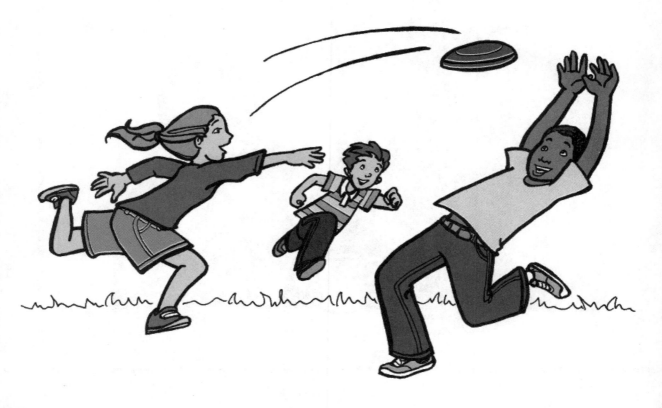

NOTE FROM THE AMA

You've reached the end of this book on puberty, but not the end of this exciting and interesting period in your life! We hope this book has answered many of your questions. Perhaps it has also encouraged you to think of even more questions. Your doctor is a good person to turn to for answers to your questions, especially if you're uncomfortable talking to other people. Keep in mind that most doctors who treat adolescents provide confidentiality—that is, they will not share information about you or things you have told them with your parents or anyone else without your permission, unless the information involves harm to you or someone else. Talk to your doctor to find out if he or she provides confidentiality.

Puberty is an exciting, strange, and wonderful process. Some of the changes you go through may seem confusing or challenging at times. Other changes make your life seem more interesting and more fulfilling. Try to enjoy this time in your life as much as you can by focusing on all the amazing things you're experiencing and accomplishing on your way to becoming an adult. Good luck!

FIND OUT MORE!...........................

For more information to help you stay healthy and safe, check out these Web sites.

BAM! BODY AND MIND

http://www.bam.gov

This site was created by the Centers for Disease Control and Prevention (CDC) to answer teens' questions about everything from health to physical education to bullying. It's also a good place to ask a question and get a helpful "Xpert opinion."

THE COOL SPOT

http://www.thecoolspot.gov/

This site offers usable information in a kid-friendly way to help kids understand the dangers of drinking alcohol. You'll also learn how to resist pressure from friends to drink.

GIRLS AND BOYS TOWN

http://girlsandboystown.org

This 24-hour national crisis hotline—800-448-3000—includes a chat room for teens in need of emergency help. It also directs visitors to counseling options in their local area.

KIDS HEALTH

http://www.kidshealth.org

This site targets many different audiences and covers many different topics. It provides extensive information to kids, including tips for staying healthy; avoiding alcohol, drugs, and cigarettes; information about eating disorders; a glossary of medical terms; and much, much more. Parents can get practical information for dealing with the many health issues affecting kids.

MIND OVER MATTER

http://www.drugabuse.gov

This excellent, informative site was developed by the National Institute on Drug Abuse. It's designed to encourage young people in grades 5 through 9 to learn about the effects of drug abuse on their body and brain.

NATIONAL ASSOCIATION OF ANOREXIA AND ASSOCIATED DISORDERS

http://www.anad.org

This is an excellent resource for people who have an eating disorder or who know someone who has one. It offers information about eating disorders and treatment centers that specialize in eating disorders. Message boards, chat rooms, and important hotline information are also available.

NATIONAL COALITION FOR GAY, LESBIAN, BISEXUAL AND TRANSGENDER YOUTH

http://www.outproud.org

This site provides information and resources for gay, lesbian, bisexual, and transgender teens, as well as for their family and friends. What is going on in schools today? Who are your community role models? Who are your peers, and how do they feel? Get answers to these questions and more at this site.

NATIONAL EATING DISORDERS ASSOCIATION

http://www.nationaleatingdisorders.org/

This site has lots of good information for both kids and parents about eating disorders: what they are, what causes them, what they can do to your body, how to recognize the signs, and how to get help.

PARTNERSHIP FOR A DRUG-FREE AMERICA

http://www.drugfree.org/Teen/

This site is loaded with information about alcohol and drugs, including steroids and inhalants. Its Help for Teens section is in a question-and-answer format to help kids understand the effects of drugs and how to get help if they or a friend has a problem.

SAFE YOUTH/NATIONAL VIOLENCE PREVENTION RESOURCE CENTER

http://www.safeyouth.org

This is a one-stop shop for information on preventing youth violence, from bullying to teen dating to violence to gang activity. This site has lots of links to other helpful sites.

STOP BULLYING NOW/HEALTH RESOURCES AND SERVICES ADMINISTRATION

http://stopbullyingnow.hrsa.gov

This government-sponsored site offers lots of fun, interactive games to help kids understand what bullying is and how to prevent it or stop it. The information is for kids who are being bullied, who witness bullying, or who bully other kids. It also provides information to adults about what they can do to help.

TALKING WITH KIDS

http://www.talkingwithkids.org

This Web site is aimed at parents, providing helpful information about how to communicate with their kids about tough issues such as sex, violence, and drugs. Although directed primarily at parents, kids can also benefit from the information.

TIPS 4 YOUTH/CENTERS FOR DISEASE CONTROL AND PREVENTION/TIPS 4 YOUTH

http://www.cdc.gov/tobacco/tips4youth.htm

This government-sponsored site provides kids with lots of information about the dangers of smoking, as well as motivation and tips for quitting. It has colorful posters and interactive animated features that appeal to kids.
about the effects of drug abuse on their body and brain.

YOUTH.ORG

http://www.youth.org

The goal of this site is to "provide young people with a safe space online to be themselves." One area on the site focuses entirely on helping young people who are questioning their sexuality. It provides many links to other sites for gay and lesbian young people.

GLOSSARY ....

This glossary defines some common terms you will find in this book. Words in italics are defined elsewhere in the glossary.

acanthosis nigricans — raised, velvety, darkened patches on the skin, often on the back of the neck, armpits, and groin, that make the skin look dirty, occurring most often in young people who are overweight

acne — a skin condition that can include *blackheads*, *whiteheads*, and/or *pimples*

Adam's apple — a bump on the front of the neck in males; is actually the front of the voicebox, or *larynx*

adolescence — the period of time during development between the end of childhood and the beginning of adulthood

AIDS — acquired immunodeficiency syndrome, the most advanced stages of infection with *HIV*

anal sex — a type of sexual activity in which an erect *penis* enters the *anus*

androgens — male *hormones*

antibiotic — a type of medicine used to treat infections caused by *bacteria*

antiperspirant — a product used to prevent perspiration or sweating

anus — the opening from which solid waste leaves the body

bacteria — microscopic organisms that can sometimes cause infection

benzoyl peroxide — a medication used to help fight *acne*

blackhead — a blemish that develops when a clogged *hair follicle* is exposed to air (referred to medically as an open comedone)

bully — a person who tries to make another person feel bad

calcium — an important *mineral* used by the body to build bones and teeth

calorie — a unit of energy the body gets from food

cancer — a disease in which abnormal cells in the body multiply and destroy healthy tissue

circumcision — removal of the *foreskin* from a *penis*

clique — a group of friends that excludes, or leaves out, other people

condom — a thin rubber or plastic covering worn on an erect penis (male condom) or inserted into the vagina (female condom) before *sex* to help prevent pregnancy and *sexually transmitted diseases*

contraceptive — a medication or device used to prevent pregnancy

cyber bullying — bullying done through the Internet

deodorant — a product that prevents or covers up unwanted odor

dermatologist — a doctor who treats skin problems

dietitian — a person who has completed a degree in nutrition and has also passed the dietitian exam

eczema — red, itchy patches on the skin that sometimes join together, occurring most often on the inner part of the elbows or behind the knees

ejaculation — the process by which *semen* leaves the body through the *penis*

epididymis — a storage area for *sperm* when they leave the *testicle*

erection — a condition in which blood fills the blood vessels and tissues of the *penis*, making it hard

flaccid — soft and limp

folliculitis — raised bumps on the skin brought on by shaving

foreskin — a fold of skin that covers the head of the *penis*

genitals — the reproductive *organs*, especially referring to those outside the body

glans — the dome-shaped head of the *penis*

growth spurt — a big increase in height in a short amount of time

hair follicle — an opening in the skin through which hair grows

heredity — the passing on of qualities and traits from one generation to the next through genetic material

hernia — a medical condition in which part of the intestine protrudes outside the wall that normally holds it (into the *scrotum*, for example*)*

HIV — human immunodeficiency syndrome, the virus that causes *AIDS*; HIV is transmitted through contact with infected blood or other body fluids, usually by having unprotected *sex* with an infected person or by sharing blood or contaminated needles

hormone — a chemical substance that controls one or more body functions

hydrocele — a buildup of fluid around the *testicles*

inflammation — the body's response to a local infection, characterized by redness, heat, swelling, and pain

jock itch — an itchy, scaly rash caused by a fungus occurring around the genital and groin areas

keloid — an abnormal, raised, hard scar that grows in an area of skin damage; some people can develop keloids after body piercings or tattoos

lacto-ovo-vegetarian — a person who does not eat meat, but whose diet includes milk and eggs

lacto-vegetarian — a person who does not eat meat, but whose diet includes milk and other dairy products

larynx — the upper part of the windpipe that contains the *vocal cords*

masturbation — stimulation of one's own *genitals* for sexual pleasure

mineral — chemicals found in foods and elsewhere; some minerals are essential for healthy functioning of the body

moles — round or oval spots on the skin that are usually dark brown and can be flat or raised

molestation — unwanted sexual touching of one person by another

nocturnal emission — *ejaculation* during sleep, also known as a *wet dream*

non-comedogenic — does not clog pores; skin products with "non-comedogenic" on the label do not contribute to the development of *acne*

nutrient — a substance required by living things to live and grow

oral sex — a type of sexual activity in which a person uses his or her mouth to stimulate another person's *genitals*

organ — a part of an animal or plant that performs one or more specific functions

orgasm — peak of sexual excitement, often accompanied by *ejaculation* in males

peer pressure — pressure from one's acquaintances, or peers, to behave in a certain way

penis — the male sex *organ*

phimosis — a medical condition in which the *foreskin* is stuck to the head of the *penis*

pimples — small areas of *inflammation* on the skin that are filled with *pus*

pink pearly papules — harmless, light-colored bumps that tend to grow in rows around the head of the *penis*; most often found in *uncircumcised* males

prostate gland — a gland surrounding the top of the *urethra* that produces a fluid that mixes with *sperm* to form *semen*

proteins — chemicals that form the structure of plants and animals; proteins in foods are essential for the body's proper growth, development, and functioning

psoriasis — patches of thick, raised skin that are pink or red and covered with silverish white scales, occurring most often on the knees, elbows, and scalp

puberty — the time during which the body grows from that of a child to that of an adult; the time during which the reproductive system matures

pubic hair — hair that grows in the genital area

pus — a creamy fluid produced as the body fights an infection

rehabilitation — strengthening exercises designed to treat sports injuries

salicylic acid — a mild acid in some medicines used to treat *acne*; it stimulates peeling of the top layer of skin and opens plugged *hair follicles*

scoliosis — a condition in which the spine curves to the left or right

scrotum — the skin sac below the *penis* that holds the *testicles*

sebum — an oily substance produced by the skin that makes the skin smooth but can also clog *hair follicles* and cause *acne*

semen — a thick, sticky, white liquid containing *sperm* cells that is ejaculated from the penis

seminal vesicles — a pair of glands on either side of the male bladder that produce a fluid that mixes with *sperm*

sex — a general term to describe sexual activities such as vaginal intercourse, *oral sex*, or *anal* sex

sexual abuse of a child — sexual mistreatment of a child, including sexual contact between an older teen or an adult and a child

sexual assault — any type of forced or unwanted sexual contact

sexual harassment — any repeated, unwanted behavior of a sexual nature performed by one person against another

sexual intercourse — when an erect *penis* enters the vagina

shaft — the part of the *penis* excluding the *glans*

smegma — a fatty, strong-smelling secretion that can collect under the *foreskin* of the *penis*

sperm — the male cell of reproduction

spermatic cords — tubes inside the *scrotum* that support the *testicles*

SPF — sun protection factor, a rating used on skin-care products to indicate the product's level of protection against sunburn

steroids — *hormones* the body produces to help the body deal with stress and promote growth and development

steroids, anabolic — versions of the male *hormone testosterone*; some athletes take artificial hormones to improve performance; when not prescribed by a physician, they are illegal and dangerous

STD — sexually transmitted disease, an infection transmitted by sexual activity

testicles — two small, oval-shaped organs that produce *testosterone* and *sperm*

testosterone — the major male sex *hormone* responsible for *sperm* production and male characteristics such as facial hair

urethra — a tube inside the *penis* that carries urine and *semen* out of the body

varicocele — a usually harmless condition in which the veins in the *scrotum* widen and stretch

vas deferens — the main tube through which *semen* travels

vegan — a person who does not eat meats, eggs, or dairy

vegetarian — a person who does not eat meat, poultry, or fish, and sometimes also avoids all animal products such as eggs and milk

vitamins — nutrients found in foods that are essential to good health

vocal cords — either of two pairs of folds in the *larynx* that vibrate and produce sound

warts — hard lumps with a rough surface that are caused by a virus, occurring most often on the arms, legs, hands, and face; planter warts develop on the bottoms of the feet; genital warts are an *STD* and occur in the genital area

wet dream — the common term for *nocturnal emission*

whitehead — a white blemish on the skin that develops when a *hair follicle* is clogged and covered and not exposed to air (referred to medically as a closed comedone)

INDEX.......................................

MEET THE MEDICAL EDITOR ....

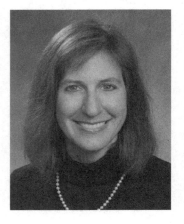

Amy B. Middleman, MD, MSEd, MPH, is a board-certified Adolescent Medicine specialist and Associate Professor of Pediatrics at Baylor College of Medicine in Houston. She is a practicing physician specializing in the care of adolescents at Texas Children's Hospital. Dr. Middleman is the Adolescent Medicine editor for the medical online text UpToDate and serves as the Society for Adolescent Medicine's liaison member of the Advisory Committee on Immunization Practices with the Centers for Disease Control and Prevention (CDC) in Atlanta. In addition to her Doctor of Medicine degree, she has a Master of Science in Education and a Master of Public Health degree.

MEET THE WRITER ....

Kate Gruenwald Pfeifer, LCSW, is a licensed clinical social worker. She has a Masters degree in social work from Columbia University as well as a certificate in psychodynamic psychotherapy with children and adolescents from NYU Psychoanalytic Institute. Pfeifer, whose practice specializing in children and adolescents is in Millburn, New Jersey, is a school social worker and supervisor of several middle school social work programs.

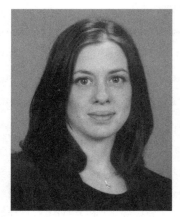

She is also the writer of the *American Medical Association's Girls's Guide to Becoming a Teen.*